NURSING MADE INSANELY EASY!

2nd Edition

Sylvia Rayfield, MN, RN, CNS
Executive Officer, I CAN, Inc.

Loretta Manning, MSN, RN, CS, GNP
Executive Officer, I CAN, Inc.

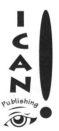

 ICAN, Inc. Publishing • Shreveport, LA

I CAN, Inc. Publishing, Shreveport, LA

P.O. Box 1135, Shreveport, Louisiana 71163 • (800) 234-0575

Editorial Assistant: Teresa R. Davidson

Cartoon Illustrations: Teresa R. Davidson, Greensboro, NC; Paulina Hanson, Words & Pictures; Jeanne Woods, Design Master, New Orleans, LA; Mitch Rubin, Rubin Art, Albuquerque, NM

Cover Design: Mason Communications, New Orleans, LA

Photographs: Griffin-Lusk Photographers, Greensboro, NC

Production: Patterson Printing, Benton Harbor, MI

Printed in the United States of America

ISBN 0-9643622-2-8

Library of Congress Catalog Card Number: 94-072947

Nursing procedures and/or practice described in this book should be applied by the nurse or healthcare practitioner under appropriate supervision according to established professional standards of care. These standards should be used with regard to the unique circumstances that apply in each practice situation. Every effort has been taken to validate and confirm the accuracy of information presented and to describe generally accepted practices. However, the authors, editors, and publisher cannot accept any responsibility for errors or omissions or for consequences from application of the information in this book and make no warranty, express or implied, with respect to the contents of this book. Every effort has been exerted by the authors and publisher to ensure that drug selection and dosage set forth in this text are in accord with current recommendations and practice at the time of publication. However, in view of ongoing research, the constant flow on information relating to governmental regulations, drug therapy, and drug reactions, the reader is urged to check the manufactures information on the package insert of each drug for any change in indications and dosage and for added warnings and precautions. This is particularly important when the recommended agent is a new or infrequently used drug. This book is written to be used as a memory tool (A Visual Approach to Memory) for students, graduates, and faculty. It is not intended for use as a primary resource for procedures, treatments, medications, or to serve as a complete textbook for nursing care. Copies of this book may be obtained directly from I CAN, Inc. (see order form in the back of this book.)

ACKNOWLEDGMENTS

We wish to express our appreciation to both our families for their never ending support and love, while we developed this book.

- Randy Manning and Betty Lynne Theriot whose strength, support, and love have been our inspiration.

- Ellis and Margaret Wright who continue to inspire us with their infinite wisdom.

- Juanita Shera who has been very inspirational and supportive with our business endeavors.

- Nancy Reynolds, our administrator and friend who always keeps us going with her vitality and enthusiasm for life.

Discovering new ways of thinking about nursing concepts is one reason for writing this book. We did not do it by ourselves. Some of these memory tools have been around for generations and we don't know their origins. Many learners and colleagues have contributed.

Marie Bremner, DSN, RN, CS
Adult Health Nursing Associate Professor,
Kennesaw State College, Marietta, GA

Jo Carol Claborn, MS, RN
Executive Director, Nursing Education Consultants, Dallas, TX

Katherine Crawford, MSN, RN
Case Manager, Quality Management,
Schumpert Medical Center, Shreveport, LA

Martha Eakes, MSN, RNC, CNA
Chair, Maternal-Neonatal Nursing,
University of North Carolina at Greensboro, Greensboro, NC

Nancy K. Lovell, MSN, RN
Medical-Surgical Nursing, Instructor of Nursing
Carl Sandburg College, Galesburg, IL

Alita R. Maddox, BSN, RN
Pediatric Nursing, Staff Nurse, PICU,
Louisiana State University, Shreveport, LA

Karna C. McBrayer, BSN, RN
Instructor, Laredo Community College, Laredo, TX

Jackie McVey, MS, RN
Assistant Professor, Northwestern State University
Division of Nursing, Shreveport, LA

Vanice W. Roberts, DSN, RN
Adult Health Nursing Professor, Chairperson of Department
of Associate Degree Nursing,
Kennesaw State College, Marietta, GA

Martha Sherman, MSN, MA, RN
Pediatric Nursing, Associate Professor,
Central Missouri State University, Warrensburg, MO

Betty Lynne Theriot, MHS, MT(ASCP), SBB
President, Creative Educators, Gulf Shores, AL

Mayola L. Villarruel, MSN, RN, CNA
Adult Health Nursing, Clinical Faculty,
Indiana University, Gary, IN

JoAnn Zerwekh, EdD, RN, CARN, CADAC, FNP
Executive Director, Nursing Education Consultants, Tucson, AZ

*Dedicated with love
to nursing students
and nursing instructors.*

I
CAN

Did is a word
　　of achievement,
Won't is a word
　　of retreat,
Might is a word
　　of bereavement
Can't is a word
　　of defeat,
Ought is a word
　　of duty,
Try is a word
　　each hour,
Will is a word
　　of beauty,
Can is a word
　　of power.

—Author Unknown

PREFACE
A Message to Our Learners

This book was developed to make life easier for student nurses in registered and practical nurse programs, medical and allied health students, new graduate nurses preparing for NCLEX-RN™ and PN™ exams, students who speak English as a second language and their respective educators.

Our experience with thousands of learners each year has helped us develop images and strategies that accelerate the learning process. The format is insanely easy! On the left page is the "bottom line stuff" about the concept. The image or memory tool is on the right page.

This 2nd edition has many additional tools to help you remember vital nursing concepts. We have added Pharmacology and the cost range of various drugs at the request of our 1st edition readers. Some of the important aspects of nursing are not easily illustrated in visuals. We think these unshown characteristics are a vital part of nursing: COMPASSION, CONSIDERATION, COLLABORATION, COMMITMENT, CALMNESS, CREATIVITY and COURAGE! We worked on this project with love and fun because we've been both student nurses and nursing teachers. We know the scope of your undertaking!

Sylvia Rayfield
Loretta Manning

"THE IMPORTANT THING IN SCIENCE IS NOT SO MUCH TO OBTAIN NEW FACTS AS TO DISCOVER NEW WAYS OF THINKING ABOUT THEM."

Sir William Bragg

COST RANGE OF MEDICATIONS

Changes in health care have made cost effectiveness mandatory. To stay marketable, the nursing profession must learn to help clients and institutions reduce costs. Currently, some institutions are giving monetary awards to nurses who intervene and identify cost effective health promotion practices in contrast to the increase in costly pharmacological agents. Drugs are a huge part of the health care cost. For these reasons we have indicated a cost range for the drugs listed in this book. This cost is not exact and is ever changing; therefore the authors and publisher can not be held accountable for total accuracy due to geographical, political, pharmaceutical, the individual ordered dosages, and other competitive factors.

We have chosen to use the "Bed and Breakfast" dollar sign ($) symbols to indicate a range. Generic costs are used when available. The authors make no judgement on the appropriateness of generic medications. Generic is simply used as a cost comparison. Over the counter drugs are often less costly than their prescription counterparts. In the back of the book there are charts with the cost ranges of the medications reviewed throughout the book. The following table may be useful when reviewing these cost ranges for medications.

$	generally under $.25 per dose
$$	range from $.26-$1.00 per dose
$$$	range from $1.01-$2.00 per dose
$$$$	range from $2.01-$3.00 per dose
$$$$$	range from $3.01-$10.00 per dose
$	megabucks! over $100.00 per dose

Our most important financial asset is our capacity to earn. Preserve and maintain to prevent limiting our options.

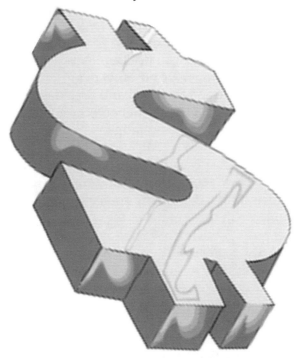

DELEGATION

The "DELEGATOR" delegates tasks but NOT responsibility. He tells his colleague how to be helpful to him. (*It is important to practice excellent communication skills or the colleague may become "stinky" like a skunk!*) Management issues are a part of the NCLEX™ Test Plan. Delegating has always been a part of management, but the scope of practice laws vary from state to state regarding the meaning of delegation. These facts are a generalization and should generally keep the DELEGATOR out of trouble on the NCLEX™. Before we **TELL** someone to do something we know that we're usually legally responsible for the outcomes. These are the facts we need to know.

T *TAUGHT*-Has the individual been taught the skill, treatment or service?

E *EVALUATE*-Just because they have been taught how to do something doesn't mean they are competent to do it. Has their return demonstration been performed and documented?

L *LICENSE*-Does the individual have or need a license to do this task? Is it within their scope of practice?

L *LISTS*-What lists of standards of care (agency policies) are written regarding this task?

Remember–The DELEGATOR delegates the task NOT THE RESPONSIBILITY!

DELEGATOR

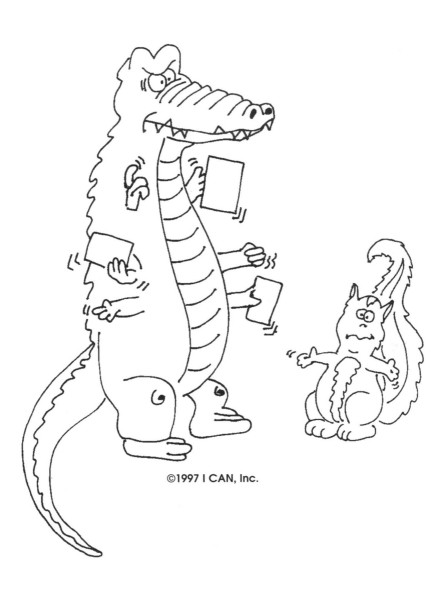

©1997 I CAN, Inc.

TABLE OF CONTENTS

HEMATOLOGIC SYSTEM

CARDIAC SYSTEM

RESPIRATORY SYSTEM

RENAL SYSTEM

REPRODUCTIVE SYSTEM

GASTROINTESTINAL SYSTEM

NEUROLOGICAL SYSTEM

MUSCULOSKELETAL SYSTEM

LABS TO REMEMBER

What we ARE communicates far more eloquently than anything we can say or do.

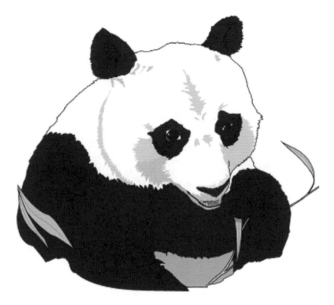

INFANCY

Check out these kids and they will help you remember milestones for these ages. Developmental task is *TRUST* versus *MISTRUST* (Erikson).

0-3 months – Recliner is in the *RECLINING* position. His head lags. At two months lifts head and chest off bed. Totally dependent. Provide toys which are soft, cuddly and colorful.

3-6 months – *SITTER* – Starts rolling over. Six months of age can SIT for short periods of time leaning forward on hands. Birth weight may double at 6 months.

6-9 months – *BOUNCER OR CRAWLER* – Can pull self to a sitting position. They start bouncing so much that they bounce out and start crawling by 8–9 months. Everything goes in the mouth. Safety precautions!

9-12 months – *CRUISER OR WALKER* – Walks with help. This age loves to cruise around furniture. The birth weight may triple and length doubled (12 months). Shows stranger anxiety; clings to mother. Continues in solitary play and can entertain self for short periods of time.

INFANCY

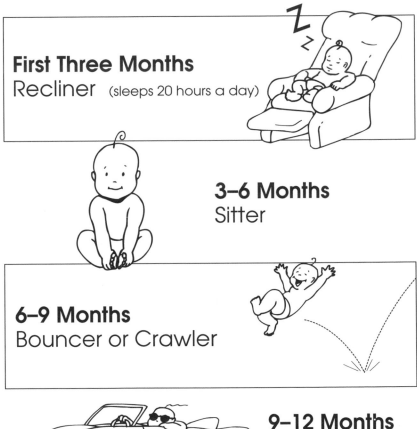

First Three Months
Recliner (sleeps 20 hours a day)

3–6 Months
Sitter

6–9 Months
Bouncer or Crawler

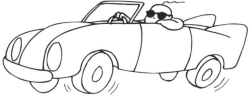

9–12 Months
Crawler or
Cruiser

©1994 I CAN

TODDLER (1 to 3 years)

These children are "Into everything," have temper tantrums, and are called the "Terrible Two's". The typical words used with the toddler are "NO NO". Let's think of the opposite and consider PRAISING positive behavior. Refer to image for this explanation.

Notice in the image the child has a *PUSH-PULL* toy which is a favorite. Anything that will make them mobile so they can be *AUTONOMOUS*. These children like playing side by side (*PARALLEL PLAY*), but forget sharing!

The **R** is for the eyes because at bed time if certain *RITUALS AND ROUTINES* are not continued they will not close their eyes and go to sleep. Moral of that story is consistency! *REGRESSION* may occur during hospitalization. **PRAISE** appropriate behavior and ignore the rest. (*Easier said than done!*)

The **A** is for the body because toddlers are into *AUTONOMY*. They like to help dress and undress self. *ACCIDENTS* are a leading cause of death. They may have bruises on extremities from climbing and *EXPLORING* (**E** for feet). Keep poisons out of reach.

The **I** is for the arms, so they can be comforted by their parents. Allow parents to stay with child to decrease those **S**'s (tears) from *SEPARATION ANXIETY*.

ELIMINATION (toilet training) is one of the major milestones for the toddler.

PRAISE

P ush-pull toys
arallel play

R ituals & routines
egression

A utonomy versus shame & doubt
ccidents

I nvolve parents

S eparation anxiety

E limination
xplore

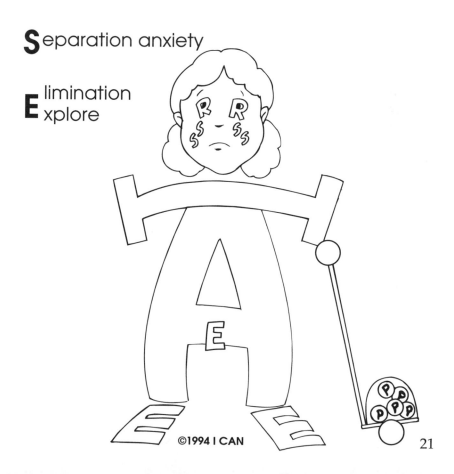

POISON CONTROL

Tommy Toxin has crawled into trouble and ingested some substance that is toxic to his body. Mom should have **Syrup of Ipecac** around the house that will make Tommy throw up the material he has ingested. Once he has vomited, **Activated Charcoal** will act as an absorbent of the poison. If he has by chance swallowed any caustic or petroleum material (i.e., kerosene, gasoline), Ipecac will be contraindicated!

Calcium EDTA a chelating agent will probably be the most effective if Tommy ate paint or has lead poisoning. Our initial focus for Tommy would be ABC's (airway, breathing, and circulation). **"POISON"** will assist you with Tommy's plan of care.

P   *PREVENT* further absorption. Decreasing absorption may be enhanced by syrup of IPECAC-in some facilities, gastric lavage has replaced Ipecac as the initial treatment. Activated charcoal may be given after gastric lavage or 30-60 minutes after induced emesis. Dialysis may be required if all else fails.

O   *OFF* - Shower or wash OFF substance if it is radioactive. If clothing is contaminated, take them OFF.
OUT - Take the toxic substance OUT of the body. If Tommy has pills in his mouth, take them OUT. Eye may need to be flushed OUT. Antidotes may be necessary for heroin or drug overdose. Ingested substances may be taken OUT of the body by emesis, lavage, absorbents, or cathartics.

I   *IDENTIFY* the toxic agent - Do an accurate history and identify any available poison.

S   *SUPPORT* the client both physically and psychologically. Parents may feel guilty in regards to their parenting role. SUPPORT is important!

O   *ONGOING* Safety education regarding poison control!

N   *NOTIFY* local poison control center, emergency facility, or physician for immediate care and advice regarding treatment.

Remember–The best solution to poisons is to keep them out of Tommy's reach!

TOMMY TOXIN

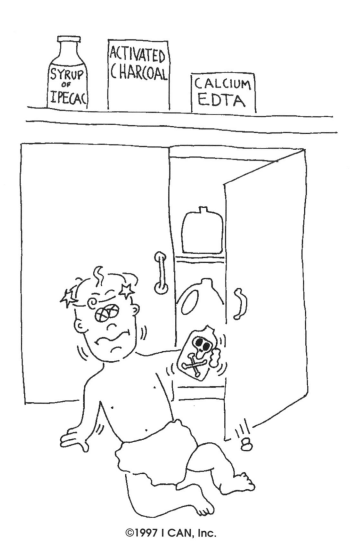

©1997 I CAN, Inc.

PRESCHOOL (3 to 6 years)

Preschoolers have imaginations that don't stop. The word that is characteristic of this stage is "Why?" They ask questions frequently. "Why is the sky blue?" "Why do dogs have tails?" Due to their active imagination, we have selected the word **MAGIC** to describe this stage of development.

M *MUTILATION*–They may fear mutilation. A typical statement is, "Cover my bo bo; don't let my blood run out!" Any invasive procedure is seen as mutilation (i.e., shot, I.V., enema, rectal temp., etc.).

A *ASSOCIATIVE PLAY*–They progress from parallel play to more cooperative play. An active imagination is great while pretending they are the nurse, doctor, teacher, etc. *ABANDONMENT*–Children are afraid of being left.

G *GUILT*–The feeling is that if I think something bad, the thought can cause a bad event to occur. This may cause guilt for the child.

I *INITIATIVE versus GUILT*–Child is very creative and may have an imaginary companion. Imaginative toys and devices are favorites.

C *CURIOUS*–Curious about factual information regarding the environment. They always ask, "Why?"

MAGIC

Mutilation

A ssociative play
bandonment

Guilt

nitiative
I maginary playmate
magination

C urious

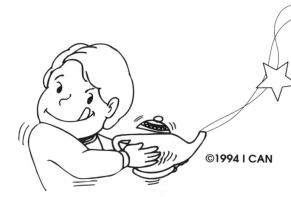

©1994 I CAN

SCHOOL AGE (6 to 12 years)

Can you see a big dimple in the chin of this child? When you look back over your school age photo albums, what do you often see in those pictures? Many of us see those crazy little **DIMPLES**!

This will help you to associate with this group.

D *DEATH*–The bogeyman will jump out from under the bed to get them. Be honest about funerals and burials. Encourage ventilation of thoughts and feelings.

I *INDUSTRY versus INFERIORITY*–"Chum" period. May enjoy collecting coins, cards, etc. May enjoy sports. *IMMUNIZATIONS* should be complete before entering school.

M *MODESTY*–More concerned with modesty and privacy. Pull those curtains and close those doors.

P *PEERS*–The younger children play mostly with their own sex. Older child is beginning to mix with opposite sex.

L *LOSS OF CONTROL*–Hospitalization is seen as a loss of control. Allow and encourage decision making.

E *EXPLAIN PROCEDURES*–Use terms they can understand.

DIMPLE

Death

Industry versus Inferiority
Immunizations

Modesty

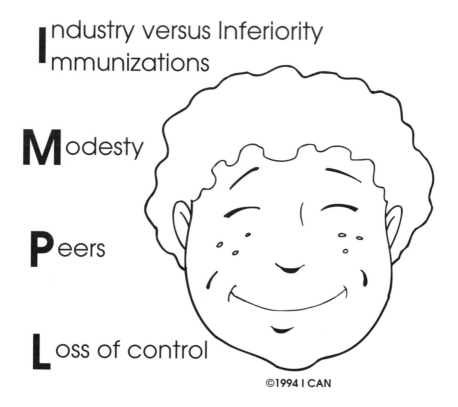

Peers

Loss of control

©1994 I CAN

Explanation of procedures

ADOLESCENT (12 to 18 years)

Adolescents are usually seen in groups or at least in **PAIRS**. Let's think about **PAIRS** while we review some milestones for the adolescent.

P   *PEER* group is very important. Select activities involving peers (i.e., games, table tennis, etc.). Remember, carefully assess the diagnosis. Individualize the plan if client is on bedrest or in isolation.

A   *ALTERED IMAGE*–They don't want to be seen as being different. Peer pressure may create problems with pregnancy, sexually transmitted diseases (STD's), substance abuse, and motor vehicle accidents. Health Promotion programs should be developed to make adolescents aware of STD's, contraception, and the effect of drugs and alcohol on the body.

I   *IDENTITY*–Adolescents may be struggling for a sense of identity. They are making important choices regarding college or career.

R   *ROLE DIFFUSION*–Who are they and what are their goals? Educate families and schools regarding these struggles.

S   *SEPARATION FROM PEERS*–Peer interaction may be encouraged during their hospitalization.

PAIRS

Peer group

Altered body image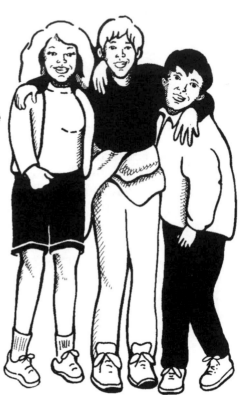

Identity—Image

Role diffusion

Separation from peers

©1994 I CAN

VITAL SIGNS

Many learners indicate they have a hard time remembering the respiratory rate and the heart rate for the various stages of development. It in reality is quite simple! All you do is start with the neonate for your guidelines.

In order to determine the respiratory rate for the toddler, subtract 10 from the neonate, and the heart rate for the toddler can be determined by subtracting 20 from the neonate. Continue in this fashion for each of the stages. The next page outlines the averages to validate your figures.

Now, was that so hard?

VITAL SIGNS

Neonate

Respiratory	40
Heart Rate	140

Toddler (age 2–4)

Respiratory	30
Heart Rate	120

Child (6–10)

Respiratory	20
Heart Rate	100

Adult

Respiratory	12–18
Heart Rate	60–100

SHOTS

Those immunizations! "Nurses think they are hot **SHOTS** giving us little babies all of those sticks!" "Let me see, what kind of complications I can develop to get those nurses to delay my **SHOTS**."

S   *SEIZURES* –"If I develop a seizure disorder, then I will not get the pertussis part of the DPT." "Second thought, that really is going to the extreme since they will go ahead with the DT."

H   *HOLD MEASLES IF EGG ALLERGY*–"I am allergic to eggs and since the measles vaccine is developed from the embryo of chicken eggs, I am certain the nurse will hold that immunization."

O   *ORGAN DEFORMITIES*–"I really do hate to develop Wilm's Tumor or cancer of any organ just to keep those nurses away from me with those shots."

T   *TEMPERATURE ELEVATED*–"The only advantage of having a fever is that my shot will not be given today."

S   *SUPPRESSED IMMUNE SYSTEM (STEROIDS)*–"If those steroids won't keep the **SHOTS** away, my suppressed immune system will. Yep, no **SHOTS** today!"

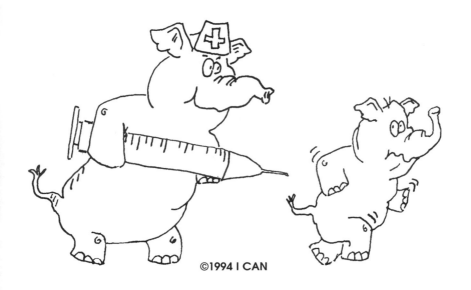

©1994 I CAN

Seizures no pertussis

Hold measles if egg allergy

Organ deformities

Temperature elevated

Suppressed immune system (steroids)

DIAGNOSTIC PROCEDURES

As you review diagnostic procedures in all areas of nursing, focus on some specific areas to maintain safety for your clients before, during and after any procedure.

We certainly do not want to "**UNDO**" any benefits from the diagnostic procedures. They are to assist with diagnostic factors–not to cause complications for the client.

U *UNDERSTAND*–Client and nurse need an understanding of the procedure. For example, a cardiac catheterization is ordered to provide data regarding status of the coronary arteries, as well as cardiac muscle function.

N *NPO*–Nothing by mouth if the procedure requires anesthesia or is invasive. The majority of gastrointestinal system diagnostics will require the client to be NPO. After a bronchoscopy, esophagoscopy or a gastroscopy, the client must remain NPO until the gag reflex returns.

D *DYES*–Assess for dye **allergy**, especially iodine and shellfish, prior to the procedure. After these procedures, fluids will be encouraged to flush the dye out of the body. Some examples of these procedures requiring dyes are myelograms, cardiac catheterizations, computerized axial tomography (CAT Scans), IVP's, etc. *Remember, the geriatric client excretes dyes slowly. Use with caution.*

P O *SITION*–Placing the client in certain POSITIONS is important during and after many procedures. This information should be part of the pretest education.

DIAGNOSTIC PROCEDURES

Understand

NPO

Dyes

p **O** sition

DANGER SIGNS IN PREGNANCY

Visualize in your mind (or on the next page) a pregnant woman who is experiencing some complications in her pregnancy. Her car will not start, and she calls a cab to take her to the hospital. The word **CABS** will help you remember these complications.

C   *CHILLS AND FEVER*–Indicative of an infection, and is never normal during pregnancy.
CEREBRAL DISTURBANCES –Headaches during pregnancy can indicate severe preeclampsia.

A   *ABDOMINAL PAIN*–Abdominal pain (epigastric area) may be due to edema of the liver capsule and may indicate a convulsion is impending. A rigid, board-like abdomen during the last trimester usually indicates abruptio placenta.

B   *BLURRED VISION*–Visual disturbances may indicate elevated *BLOOD PRESSURE* or a complication with severe preeclampsia.
BLEEDING–Early bleeding could indicate a miscarriage, abortion, ectopic pregnancy or hydatiform mole. Bleeding in the last trimester may be indicative of placenta previa or abruptio placenta.

S   *SWELLING*– Edema especially in the periorbital and digital areas is indicative of mild preeclampsia. Watch for *SUDDEN ESCAPE OF FLUID* (rupture of membranes)!

DANGER SIGNS IN PREGNANCY

C hills and fever
erebral disturbances

A bdominal pain

B lurred vision
lood pressure
leeding

S welling
udden escape of fluid

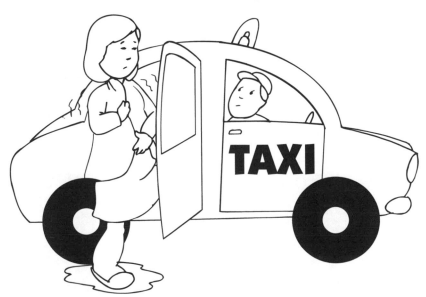

PREECLAMPSIA

Pregnancy-induced hypertension (PIH) is the term used for hypertensive disorders specifically associated with pregnancy, preeclampsia and eclampsia. Our objective with this tool is to identify the mild signs and severe signs with preeclampsia.

MILD PREECLAMPSIA– The triad of symptoms for PIH are:

> *HYPERTENSION*–Systolic increase of 30 mm Hg. and diastolic increase of 15 mm Hg. over baseline.

> *EDEMA*–Generalized digital and periorbital edema. Weight gain of 1 lb./week in 3rd trimester.

> *PROTEINURIA*–1 gm/24 hours (1+ protein).

SEVERE PREECLAMPSIA–The diagram illustrates the signs of severe preeclampsia. Add the signs of mild with severe to complete the severe assessments.
- Epigastric pain (due to liver edema) usually indicates an impending convulsion.

PREECLAMPSIA

MILD

Hypertension

Edema

Proteinuria

SEVERE

Cerebral

Visual

Vomiting

Epigastric

Oliguria

PREGNANCY-INDUCED HYPERTENSION

This condition is specifically associated with pregnancy, preeclampsia and eclampsia. When you think about the priority nursing care with this disorder, think about **PEACE**. It is of paramount importance to provide a peaceful environment to prevent seizure activity.

P *PROMOTE BEDREST, QUIET ENVIRONMENT*–These are crucial. In severe preeclampsia, absolute bedrest and sedatives (Valium) are important.

E *ENSURE HIGH PROTEIN INTAKE*–Due to proteinuria, protein intake should be increased in the diet. Sodium intake should remain normal. Avoid diuretics.

A *ANTIHYPERTENSIVE DRUGS*–Apresoline is a vasodilator that may be used to decrease the blood pressure. It's safe since it doesn't cross the placental membrane. Check maternal BP, pulse and FHR.

C *CONVULSIONS*–Prevent or control seizures. Administer IV Magnesium Sulfate. Have the antidote, calcium gluconate at the bedside for emergencies. Decrease the environmental stimuli.

E *EVALUATE PHYSICAL PARAMETERS*–Evaluate for complications of magnesium sulfate toxicity.

PREGNANCY-INDUCED HYPERTENSION

Promote bedrest,
    quiet environment

Ensure high protein intake
    (1g/kg/day)

Antihypertensive drug:
    Hydralazine (Apresoline)

Convulsions (Magnesium Sulfate)

Evaluate physical parameters

1. Blood pressure
2. Urine output
3. Respirations
4. Patella reflex

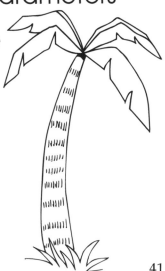

MAGNESIUM SULFATE TOXICITY

Magnesium Sulfate is the drug given to women to prevent seizures with the complication of pregnancy-induced hypertension (PIH). This medicine is a central nervous system depressant. The antidote is calcium gluconate. How can you remember the signs of too much of this medicine? Just remember that before a client has a seizure they may let out a loud **BURP**! (Do they do this in reality? Not usually; it is only a memory technique.)

Let me introduce you to Bonnie Burp. She has the following problems:

B *BLOOD PRESSURE DECREASED*

U *URINE OUTPUT DECREASED*

R *RESPIRATIONS DECREASED*

P *PATELLA REFLEX ABSENT*

Bonnie is predisposed to these side effects because magnesium sulfate is a central nervous system depressant. It acts by blocking the neuromuscular transmission.

MAGNESIUM SULFATE TOXICITY

Blood pressure decreased

Urine output decreased

Respirations < 12

Patella reflex absent

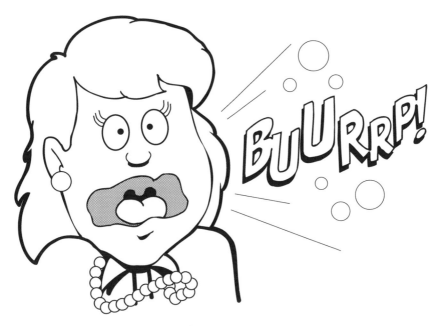

©1994 I CAN

NONSTRESS TEST–OBSTETRICAL DIAGNOSTIC TEST

The purpose of this test is to observe the *RESPONSE* of the fetal heart rate to the stress of activity.

Procedure requires approximately 30 minutes; mother is in semi-Fowler's position; external monitor is applied to document fetal activity; mother activates the "mark button" on the electronic fetal monitor when she feels fetal movement.

NONREACTIVE
NONSTRESS
NOT GOOD

REACTIVE
   (Rate of heart is elevated in response to stress of activity)
RESPONSE IS
REAL GOOD from nonstress test

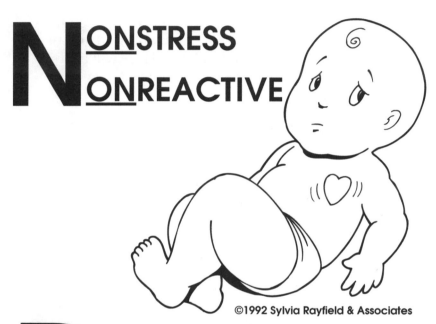

NONSTRESS

NONREACTIVE

©1992 Sylvia Rayfield & Associates

REACTIVE

RESPONSE IS

REAL GOOD

SIGNS AND SYMPTOMS OF LABOR AND DELIVERY

Would you agree with us if we say there is a fetus in the uterus wanting to be delivered into the **WORLD**? The fetus will go through the mechanisms of labor. There will be some signs that will indicate this process is imminent. The word **"WORLDS"** will help.

W *WEIGHT LOSS* –Nausea, vomiting, diarrhea and indigestion are responsible for this sign.

O *OBSERVE CHANGE IN SENSATIONS* –Since lightening, the mother may no longer have shortness of breath. Now she may experience some rectal pressure and an increase
in the leg cramps.

R *RUPTURE OF THE MEMBRANES* –After membranes rupture, delivery should occur within 24 hours to minimize the risk of infection.

L **LIGHTENING**–This is when the fetus descends into the pelvis. Mothers will refer to this as their baby "dropping."

D *DILATION AND EFFACEMENT*–These are the most indicative signs that labor is pending. Dilation is when the cervix progresses from 0 to 10 cm. in diameter, and effacement is the thinning of the cervix.

S *SHOW BLOODY*– This is the expulsion of the mucous plug.

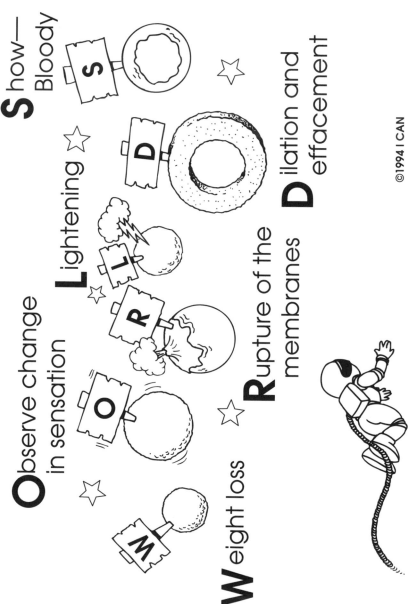

Weight loss

Observe change in sensation

Lightening

Rupture of the membranes

Show—Bloody

Dilation and effacement

©1994 I CAN

47

MECHANISMS OF LABOR AND DELIVERY

How does that fetus get through the birth canal? Can you remember the sequence of events off the top of your head? If you can remember the following jingle, you will be able to easily recall the mechanisms.

EVERY DARN FOOL IN EGYPT EATS RAW EGGS.

Take the first letter of each of these words, and you will be able to come up with the order of mechanisms. (Refer to the next page for the exact order.)

MECHANISMS OF LABOR

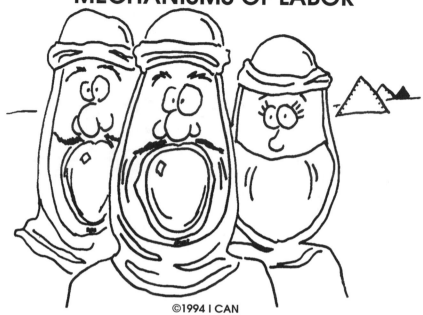

©1994 I CAN

Every	=	**E**ngagement
Darn	=	**D**escent
Fool	=	**F**lexion
In	=	**I**nternal Rotation
Egypt	=	**E**xtension
Eats **R**aw	=	**E**xternal **R**otation
Eggs	=	**E**xpulsion

DECELERATIONS

What is happening? As you can see on the next page, there is pressure on the head of the fetus. The difference in this *EARLY DECELERATION* in contrast to a *LATE DECELERATION* is that the onset, fall and recovery of the heart rate coincide with the onset, peak and end of the contraction. This does not indicate a problem and usually occurs during the active phase of labor.

LATE DECELERATIONS indicate a problem with uteroplacental insufficiency. (Refer to **LATE DECELERATIONS.**)

VARIABLE DECELERATIONS are usually shaped like a V or a squared U. These may occur any time during the contraction cycle or may be nonrepetitive. The pathophysiology is cord compression. The nursing care is to change the position of the mother. If it lasts more than one minute, attempt upward displacement of presenting part. Mother may be placed in the knee-chest position or Trendelenburg position. This pattern may indicate a prolapsed cord. If this is the case, prepare for immediate delivery. To assist with fetal oxygenation, the nurse may give the mother oxygen.

DECELERATIONS

head compression

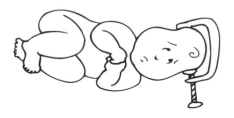

Early

Late

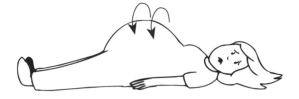

---

cord compression

Variable

LATE DECELERATIONS

The Fire Department has come to the rescue of **FETAL DIS-TRESS**, and is planning to put out the problem. First, however, they must **UNCOIL** the fire hose. What does a late deceleration look like and what does it mean? It is a uniform shaped dip. The onset coincides with the peak of the contraction with the recovery occurring at the end or after the end of the contraction. It indicates uteroplacental insufficiency. If the fire department does not do something soon, the fetus is going to get into severe distress.

C   *CHANGE POSITION*–Place mother in the left lateral position. For supine hypotension, change the maternal position.

O   *OXYGEN*–Administer oxygen to mother to correct the uteroplacental insufficiency. If *OXYTOCIN* is infusing, stop the infusion. This may be causing uterine hyperactivity resulting in uteroplacental insufficiency.

I   *IV FLUIDS*–Epidurals may cause dilation. Increasing hydration with IV fluids will increase the maternal blood pressure and the uteroplacental circulation.

L   *LOWER THE HEAD OF THE BED* and elevate the feet to increase perfusion to the uterus.

LATE DECELERATIONS

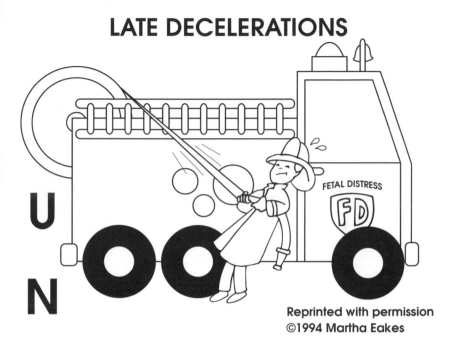

FETAL DISTRESS

FD

Reprinted with permission
©1994 Martha Eakes

U
N

C hange position (left side)

O xygen
xytocin—off

I V fluids

L ower head

ACTIVE PHASE

During the first phase of labor, the mother is extroverted, feels great, and is going natural childbirth all the way (until she gets to this second phase)! Now, life has changed, and she is down right **MAD**! During the active phase of labor, mother is 4-7 cm. dilated with contractions occurring every 3-5 minutes lasting for 30-60 seconds. This phase can last approximately 6 hours.

M *MEDICATIONS* – Have the meds ready! She may reconsider and have an epidural. Meds are not given in the first phase (Latent) because they may slow the progress of labor. They are not given during the third phase due to potential suppression of the neonatal respiratory status.

A *ASSESS* – Assessments include: vital signs, cervical dilation and effacement, fetal monitor, etc.
ANTICIPATE PHYSICAL NEEDS–Mothers will appreciate you sponging their face, keeping their LINENS clean and DRY. Assess bladder for fullness.

D *DRY LIPS* – Mouth gets dry and can crack. Provide oral care! Mom will love you for being so thoughtful. (It's the little things that really count!)

ACTIVE = 4-7 cm.

q 3-5 min. contractions
30-60 seconds duration

Medications

Assess
nticipate physical needs

Dry lips—ointment
ry linens

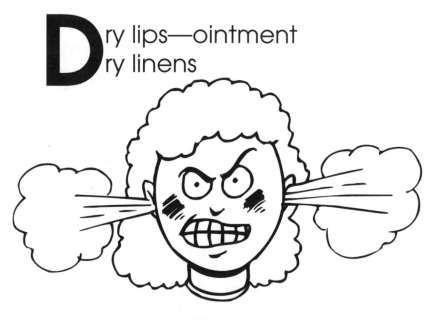

PITOCIN

Pitty Pitocin, this pregnant woman, is slow to begin active labor, so the Doc decides to induce by using **PITOCIN**. Watch for those major side effects!

Visualize Pitty sitting in a row boat looking into a **PIT** watching the "TETANIC" sink into the "ocean" (**OCIN**). Complications of this drug are **TETANIC CONTRACTIONS**. Pitocin of course is a stimulant; so as Pitty watches the ship sink, her blood *PRESSURE* elevates! Just as a sinking ship takes in all that salty WATER, poor Pitty is left holding the excess fluid in her body (observe **INTAKE and OUTPUT**). She gets so nervous with all this happening that she goes into **CARDIAC ARRHYTHMIAS** causing Pitty's baby *OXYGEN* hunger and FETAL HEART **IRREGULARITIES**. This is so upsetting to Pitty that she gets *NAUSEATED* and **VOMITS** all over the row boat.

STOP THAT PITOCIN DRIP!!!!!!

SIDE EFFECTS OF PITOCIN

Pressure is elevated

Intake and output

Tetanic contractions

Oxygen decrease in fetus

Cardiac arrhythmia

Irregularity in fetal heart rate

Nausea and vomiting

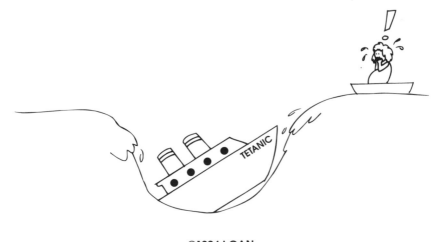

©1994 I CAN

ANESTHESIA

Regional anesthesia is used to anesthetize one **REGION** of the body; the client may remain awake and alert throughout the procedure. The image used will assist in recalling nursing care for the different **REGIONS** of the body.

R *RESPIRATORY PARALYSIS* – Have ventilatory support equipment available. Avoid the extreme Trendelenburg position before level of anesthesia is set.

E *ELIMINATION* – Evaluate the bladder for distention. When the epidural is done on a pregnant woman, labor may be delayed due to bladder distention.

G *GASTROINTESTINAL* – Check when client last ate. Position to prevent aspiration. Antiemetics need to be available along with suction equipment.

I *INFORM OF PROCEDURE* – Does the client understand the procedure? Check for drug allergies, make sure legal permit is signed and have client empty bladder.

O *OBSERVE FOR HYPOTENSION* – Report B/P less than 100 systolic, or any significant decrease. Change client's position, administer oxygen and increase IV rate if client is not prone to CHF.

N *NO TRAUMA TO EXTREMITIES* – Support extremities during movement. Remove legs from stirrups together.

ANESTHESIA

Respiratory paralysis

Elimination

GI

Inform of procedure

Observe for hypotension

No trauma to the extremities

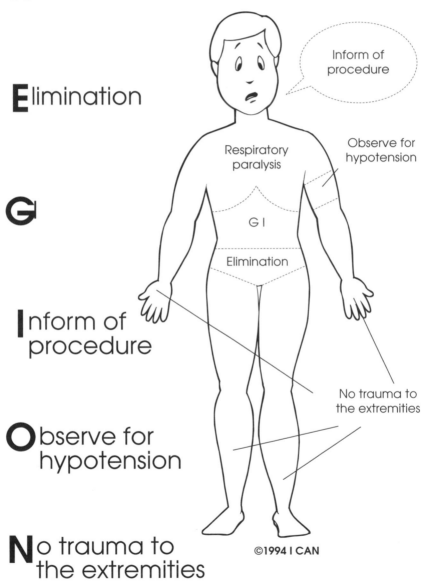

TRANSITIONAL

This is the last phase of the first stage of labor. Mother has gone from being MAD to being **TIRED**. She is now 8-10 cm. dilated and contractions are occurring every 2-3 minutes, lasting 45-90 seconds. This exhausting phase has duration of 1-2 hours. (MUCH TOO LONG; MOTHERS SAY!)

T *TIRES*–The mother continues to need a great deal of physical and emotional support.

I *INFORM OF PROGRESS*–Time drags on during this phase! The smallest progress is important.

R *RESTLESS*– "Please, can we get this show on the road?" (We were being polite; most mothers forget the word please at the peak of a contraction.) Support mothers with their breathing techniques. We don't want her pushing until she is totally dilated, so short panting breaths would be appropriate here.

E *ENCOURAGE AND PRAISE*–Go for it!

D *DISCOMFORT*–Mom is going to put all of her negotiating skills to work here in order to get the nurse to give her some pain medicine. No analgesics are given here because of the effect on the neonate's respiratory status.

TRANSITIONAL = 8-10 cm.

q 2-3 min. contractions
45-90 seconds duration

Tires

Inform of progress

Restless

Encourage and praise

Discomfort

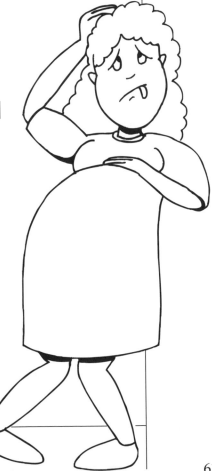

POSTPARTUM ASSESSMENT

If a parent's newborn is a son, they must "BUBBLE HE" during and after feedings. This will assist you with reviewing the postpartum assessment.

B *BREAST*–Assess for and prevent mastitis. Teach how to cleanse breasts and nipples. Support with breast feeding.

U *UTERUS*–Fundus should be firm and in the midline. Immediately after delivery, the top of the fundus is several finger breadths above the umbilicus. The fundus then descends into the pelvis approximately one finger breadth per day. Massage the fundus if it is boggy.

B *BLADDER*–Observe for bladder distention; it may displace the uterus. Diuresis occurs during the first two postpartal days. Evaluate for UTI.

B *BOWEL*–Stool softeners or laxatives may be necessary. By second or third day post delivery, normal bowel movements should occur.

L *LOCHIA*–Should not have foul odor. Rubra (dark red first 3 days), serosa (pinkish, sero-sanguinous 3 -10 days) and alba (creamy or yellowish after 10th day and may last a week or two).

E *EPISIOTOMY*–Observe for infection and healing.

H *HOMAN'S SIGN*–Observe for thrombophlebitis.

E *EMOTIONAL*–Support is a must!

POSTPARTUM ASSESSMENT

B reast

U terus

B ladder

B owel

L ochia

E pisiotomy

H oman's sign

E motional

Reprinted with permission
©1994 Martha Eakes

FOLIC ACID

Several conditions require a client to eat a diet high in folic acid. Some examples of these are: iron deficiency anemia, chronic alcoholism in a pregnant mother and malnutritional anemia. Here is a visual to help you remember those foods high in Folic Acid.

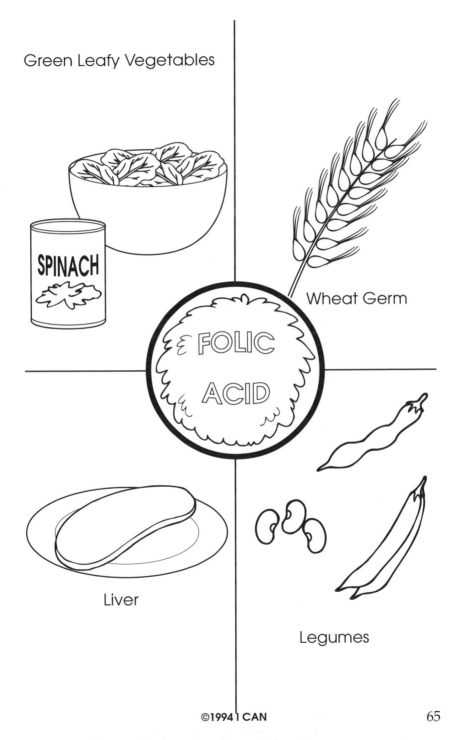

Green Leafy Vegetables

SPINACH

Wheat Germ

FOLIC ACID

Liver

Legumes

FOODS HIGH IN IRON

What type of clients need to be on a diet high in iron? If you indicated any of the following, you are right. Clients with hemodilutional anemia who are pregnant, poor dietary intake of iron, surgery of gastrointestinal tract, problems with absorption and clients on IV therapy for 10 days or more need to be on a diet high in iron.

The foods which are high in iron are: organ meats (think about an organ that plays music), red meats, fish, green leafy vegetables, raisins (the California Raisin), sunflower seeds and legumes.

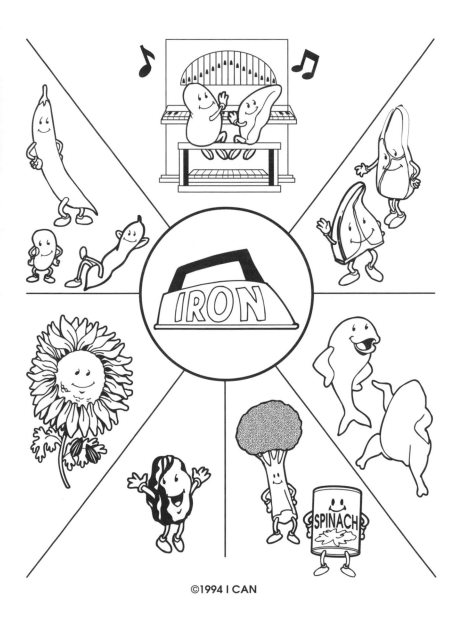

©1994 I CAN

FOODS HIGH IN PROTEIN

Foods high in protein can easily be remembered if you recall the jingle *Happy To Consume My Calories Sanely*. **H**amburger, **T**una, **C**hicken, **M**ilk, **C**ottage Cheese and **S**oy Beans are high in protein.

PROTEIN

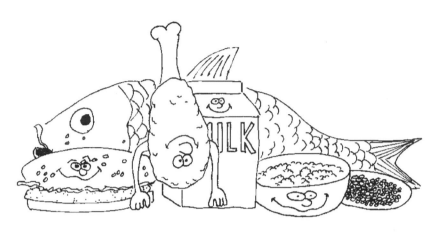

©1994 I CAN

Happy	=	**H**amburger
To	=	**T**una
Consume	=	**C**hicken
My	=	**M**ilk
Calories	=	**C**ottage Cheese
Sanely	=	**S**oy Beans

FOODS HIGH IN POTASSIUM

An easy way to remember foods high in Potassium (K$^+$) is the **ABC Fruit** and **Veggie Plate**. Apples, Bananas, Cantaloupe (melons) and Citrus such as orange juice are high in K$^+$. Asparagus, Broccoli and Carrots are also high in potassium. Teach clients about the **ABC Fruit** and **Veggie Plate**, especially those clients who are taking diuretics.

Clients with severe burns, others who have hypersecretion of the adrenal cortex or on long term steroid therapy will benefit from these foods.

K FOODS = ABC FRUIT/VEGGIE PLATE

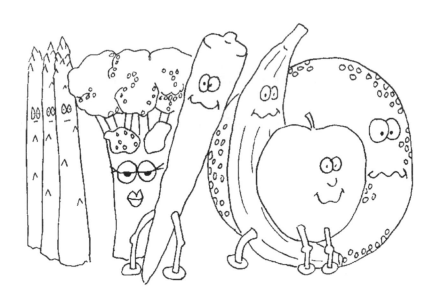

©1994 I CAN

FRUITS
Apples
Bananas
Cantaloupe

VEGGIES
Asparagus
Broccoli
Carrots

FOODS HIGH IN SODIUM

The all-American **HOT DOG**–your way to remember foods that are high in salt (sodium). What is the first thing you must have for a hot dog? A wiener of course. Can't have a hot dog without a wiener and what is a wiener? It's processed meat in a tube that is high in salt.

Now, imagine walking through the delicatessen with us, looking up and seeing all of those tubes of meat hanging from the ceiling. Pressed ham, salami, bologna–all high in salt. Next we need a bun for the wiener. Of course, we put baking soda in our bread to make it rise (soda is salt). Next, comes ketchup which is processed tomatoes that are high in salt. Some folks will mess up a perfectly good hot dog with pickles! Did you ever make pickles? You throw cucumbers into brine (salt water). Those who have to have a chili dog, open a can of chili. Canned foods are usually high in salt. Then of course some of our German friends must have sauerkraut on their dogs which is also high in salt. So, to remember those foods high in sodium, all you have to know is **HOT DOG**!

FOODS HIGH IN SODIUM

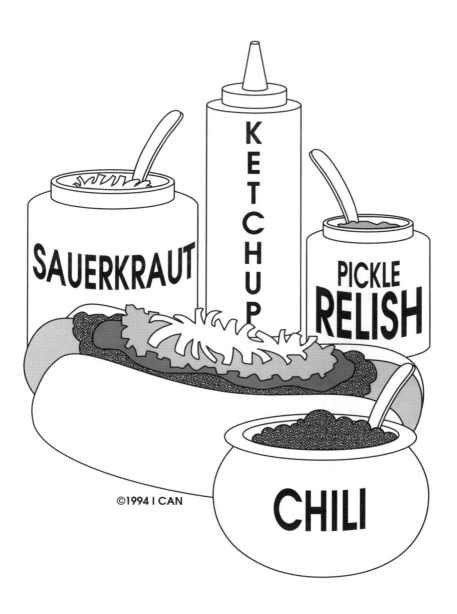

©1994 I CAN

LOW RESIDUE DIET

Daddy had some sort of rectal surgery or diarrhea that makes it a necessity for him to sit on his pillow. Low residue diets are used to reduce fiber and slow bowel movements. Clients with Crohn's disease and colitis may benefit from this particular diet. Here's an easy way to remember the low residue diet.

L   *LIMITED FAT AND FRIED FOODS*

O   *ZERO MILK*

R   *REAL FRESH FISH / UNSEASONED GROUND MEAT*

E   *EGGS BOILED*, not fried

S   *STRAINED FOODS*

As you can see for yourself, this diet is NO FUN for Daddy!

LOW RESIDUE DIET

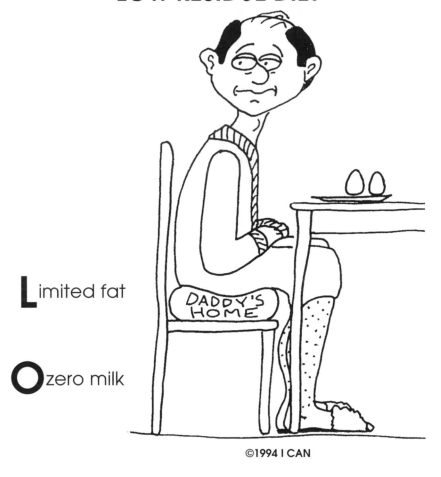

Limited fat

Ozero milk

©1994 I CAN

Real fresh fish/ground meat

Eggs boiled

Strained foods

75

TRUST

Therapeutic interaction takes place when **TRUST** is established. Think of joining hands with someone special to you. The letters in **TRUST** help us remember the dynamics of therapeutic communication.

T *TRY EXPRESSION*–Encourage the exploration of thoughts, perceptions, feelings, and actions. Use broad openings and ask open ended questions.

R *REFLECTION OF WORDS*–Confirms to the person that you are actively listening. For example, "I am really mad at my mother for grounding me." "You sound angry because you were grounded."

U *USE OF SILENCE*–Just sit and allow the person to make the next response.

S *SETTING LIMITS*–What type of people may need to have limits set? People with personality and substance abuse disorders, affective disorders, children and spouses.

T *TIME WITH CLIENT*–Taking time with the client allows them to know that you care even if they refuse to communicate.

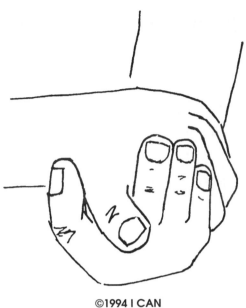

©1994 I CAN

Try expression

Reflection of words

Use of silence

Set limits

Time with client

EATING DISORDERS

Our friend, Hortense , has a major eating disorder. These disorders consist of anorexia nervosa, bulimia or pica. Hortense has bulimia, recurrent episodes of binge eating. Anorexia is an intense fear of becoming obese. Pica is persistent eating of substances without nutritional value such as clay for at least one month.

So what is the bottom line problem? It is a feeling of loss of control and low self-esteem. Let's look at **EATING** to help remember.

E *ENCOURAGE EXPRESSION OF FEELINGS*–Help identify angry and negative feelings and recognize her positive characteristics.

A *ALWAYS USE THE SAME SCALES* –Weigh daily immediately upon arising and following first voiding.

T *TO PROMOTE FEELINGS OF CONTROL*, encourage independent decision making.

I *INCLUDE DIETITIAN* and Hortense to determine calories required. Once the plan is developed do not discuss food or eating.

N *NO SIGNS OF MALNUTRITION*–Observe amount of food ingested. Offer support and positive reinforcement for improvements in eating behaviors.

G *GOAL*–To identify eating disorder and rule out physiological etiology. *Assist Hortense to re-examine self and identify positive characteristics.*

HAVE PATIENCE!

EATING DISORDERS

Encourage expression of feelings

Always use the same scales

To promote feelings of control

Include dietitian

No signs of malnutrition

Goal

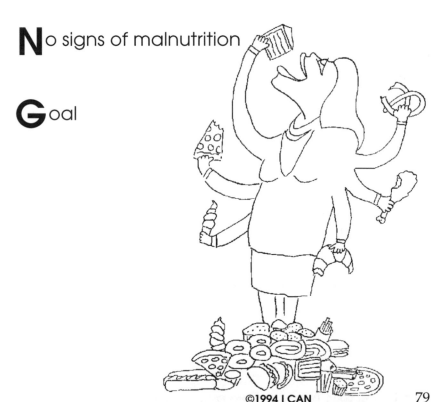

INTERVENTIONS FOR ANXIETY

ANXIETY! Welcome to nursing school! Would you agree? Perhaps we should say, "Welcome to life!" Before we can successfully help our clients deal with their anxiety, we need to remain **CALMER** ourselves.

C *CALM*–Create a comfortable, calm environment for relaxation. A quiet room with soft music may help enhance this feeling.

A *AWARENESS OF ANXIETY* – Identify and describe feelings. Modify stress producing situations.

L *LISTEN*–Listen to both client and to yourself. Implement "TRUST." Protect the defenses and coping mechanisms.

M *MEDICATIONS*–When all else fails, use those drugs. A memory tool for anti-anxiety medications is on the next page.

E *ENVIRONMENT*–Walking, crying, working and concrete tasks may help moderate anxiety. Safety is paramount if meds have to be used.

R *REASSURANCE* –Implement "TRUST."

INTERVENTIONS FOR ANXIETY

Calm

Anxiety-aware

Listen

Meds—Librium, Equanil, Atarax, Valium, and Serax

Environment

Reassurance

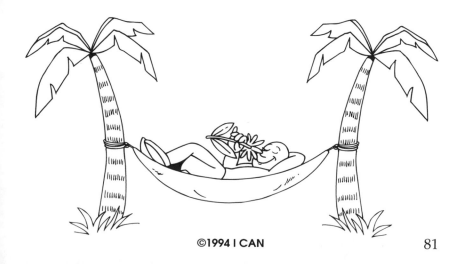

ANTI-ANXIETY MEDICINES

To stay calmer, smell the flowers in life. What are on flowers? Leaves are on flowers. If you take the first letter of each of the letters in "**LEAVS**" it will help you remember these medicines. Yes, we know "**LEAVS**" is not spelled correctly, but it will help get the point across.

L   *LIBRIUM*–Reduces anxiety. Teach not to drink alcohol while taking any anti-anxiety agent or abruptly stop taking these medications. Watch for signs of leukopenia such as sore throat, fever and weakness. Teach client to rise slowly to reduce postural hypotension.

E   *EQUANIL*–Action is similar to Librium and Valium (BENZODIAZEPINES). Metabolizes extensively in the liver and interferes with liver function tests. Decreases PT if on coumadin.

A   *ATARAX*–Does not cause tolerance and can be used temporarily when other anti-anxiety agents have been abused.

V   *VALIUM*–Same actions, side effects and nursing implications as Librium.

S   *SERAX*–Useful for treating elderly clients. Does not rely on liver for metabolism.

ANTI-ANXIETY MEDICINES

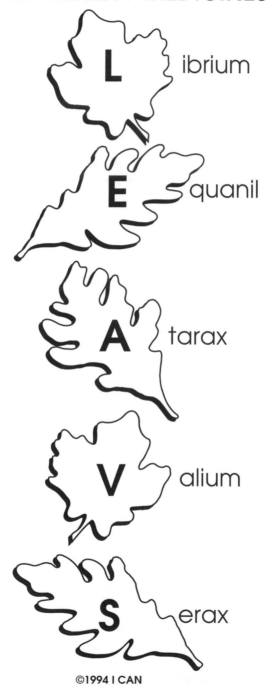

L ibrium

E quanil

A tarax

V alium

S erax

DEPRESSION

A depressed individual reminds us of a FLAT tire with all the air depressed out. When you think about the assessments for the depressed client, let's think of a "**FLAT**" tire.

F *FLAT AFFECT*–A face without an expression.

L *LETHARGIC*–Feelings of fatigue, lack of appetite, constipation, sleeping disturbances (insomnia or early morning wakefulness), decrease in libido. Despairing, loss of interest or pleasure in most usual activities.

A *APATHY*–Repressed guilt can lead to apathy and feelings of helplessness and hopelessness.

T *TEARFUL*–Negative view of self, world and of the future; poverty of ideas; crying and suicidal preoccupation. This can occur as a result of turning aggressive feelings inward and displacing them onto self; accompanied by feelings of guilt.

DEPRESSION

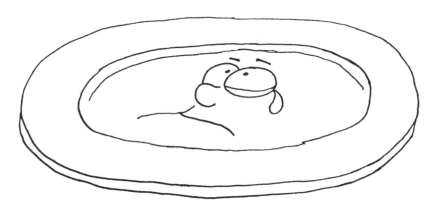

©1994 I CAN

ASSESSMENT:

Flat affect

Lethargic

Apathy

Tearful

MANAGEMENT OF DEPRESSION

The depressed client is frequently seen alone and withdrawn from any meaningful social activities. The ultimate goal is to restore that socialization. Before that can be accomplished, trust with the nurse and eventually trust with a "**PEER**" must be established.

P   *PREVENT SUICIDE*–The presence of a suicidal plan, including specifics relating to the method all indicate a potential risk. Remove harmful objects.

E   *ENVIRONMENT*–A structured environment usually works best for the depressed client due to their impairment in decision-making. Encourage participation in activities and other simple tasks.

E   *ESTEEM*–Encourage activities that promote a sense of accomplishment and enhance self-esteem. Encourage exercise and adequate rest.

R   *RELATIONSHIP*–Encourage expression of feelings, thoughts or depressed feelings. Convey a kind, pleasant, concerned approach to promote a sense of dignity and self-worth in the client.

MANAGEMENT OF DEPRESSION

Prevent suicide

Environment

Esteem

Relationships

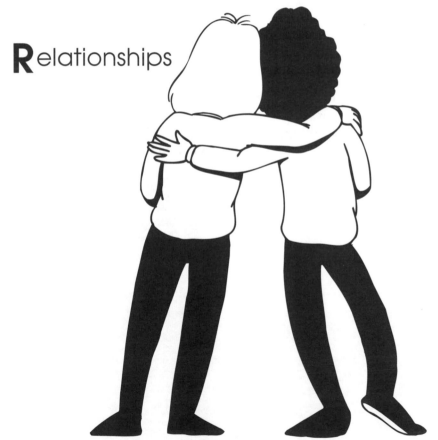

ANTIDEPRESSANTS - TRICYCLICS

Some of these medications can be recalled if you remember the jingle **EACH VICTIM'S A TOUGH NEUROTIC**. Take the first letter of each word (including the **S** in *VICTIM'S*), and this will assist you with this process. *ELAVIL, VIVACTIL, SINE-QUAN, AVENTYL, TOFRANIL, AND NORPRAMIN.*

TRICYCLICS

Each	=	**E**lavil
Victim'**S**	=	**V**ivactil **S**inequan
A	=	**A**ventyl
Tough	=	**T**ofranil
Neurotic	=	**N**orpramin

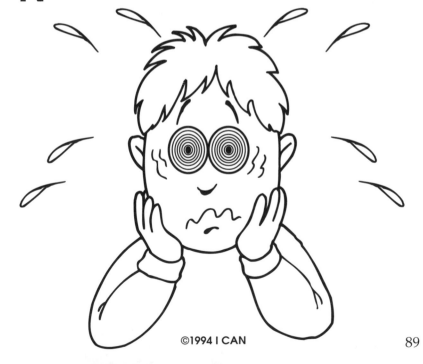

MONOAMINE OXIDASE INHIBITORS (MAO)

A few examples of these antidepressant medications are Marplan, Nardil and Parnate. They are given to inhibit the enzyme, monoamine oxidase, which breaks down norepinephrine and serotonin, increasing the concentration of these neurotransmitters. To assist you in reviewing the foods to stay away from while on these medicines, refer to the king on the next page or think of a tyrant (representing tyramine).

At 4:30 P.M. he goes into his study, and sits down to an ice cold mug of BEER, 2 glasses of WINE, and a platter of aged CHEESE. Later on in the evening, he goes into his dining room for a plate of LIVERS, home made steaming hot YEAST ROLLS, a bowl of FIGS, a glass of COLA, and a large piece of CHOCOLATE pie. In the middle of the table, there are 7 bottles of OVER-THE-COUNTER COLD MEDICINES. Tyramine is in most of these.

If the client takes tyramine (or any of these foods or meds), while on the MAO, it will cause a HYPERTENSIVE CRISIS. This will be characterized by increased temperature, tremors, tachycardia and a marked elevation in the blood pressure.

Watch for Strokes!

MONOAMINE OXIDASE (MAO) INHIBITORS

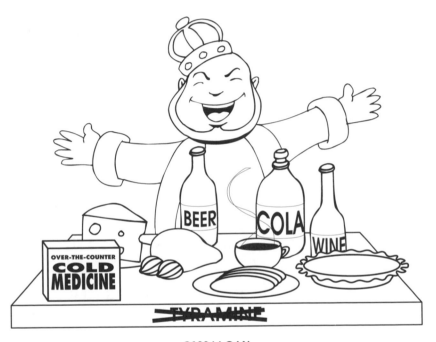

©1994 I CAN

BIPOLAR DISORDER

This psychiatric challenge is very well named. Our clown is interestingly dressed on one side and quite shabbily dressed on the other. Unless these folks are treated, their behavior is at opposite ends of the pole. Sometimes they will be so **UP** that they are manic, and other times they are so **DOWN** in the dumps that they're ready to kill themselves.

When they are **UP**, they may think they are Elvis or some other magnificent person. They may think this 24 hours a day. They don't have time to rest, eat or sleep. Try giving them finger foods and providing noncompetitive activities to decrease their hyperactivity. Setting limits, being firm and helping them stay on Detakote or Lithium may be the best approach. Lithium works best when there is a sodium balance, so try to find them something to do besides play football which is sure to make them sweat. (Besides, this is competitive–Talk about hyper!)

When they are **DOWN**, it's hard to please them. Everything is negative, nothing is right. They still do not eat or sleep well because they are too depressed. Suicide is a common problem. Maintain Lithium at 0.5-1.5 meq/L. Report any assessment which will alter the sodium level.

GOOD LUCK!

BIPOLAR DISORDER

Mood elevated

A grandiose delusion

Need for sleep, eat ↓

Inappropriate

Clanging, loud, vulgar

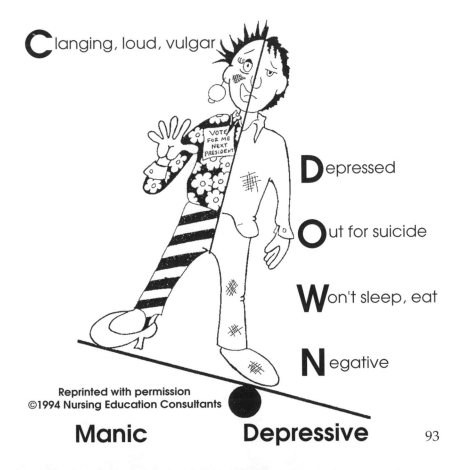

Depressed

Out for suicide

Won't sleep, eat

Negative

Manic   **Depressive**

93

LITHIUM

Lithium is used for the **manic** episode in biplolar disorder. It acts to lower concentrations of norepinephrine and serotonin by inhibiting their release. Maintenance lithium serum levels should be between .5 - 1.5 mEq / Liter. Blood tests need to initially be done weekly. Maintenance blood **levels** should be done one time per month. Lithium should be taken the same time each day preferably with meals or milk. Do not crush, chew, or break the extended - release or film coated tablets.

Laboratory studies of the **thyroid** hormone and periodic palpation of the thyroid gland should be a part of preventive therapy. Report signs of hypothyroidism. Symptoms are reversible when lithium is discontinued and supplemental thyroid is provided.

Polyuria or **incontinence**, mild **thirst**, fine **hand tremors** or jaw tremors may occur in early treatment of mania or some-times persist throughout therapy. Usually however, symptoms subside with temporary reduction of dose. A neuromuscular reaction is
unsteady gait.

Encourage a diet containing normal amounts of **salt** and a **fluid** intake of 3 liters per day. Assess clients who are high risk to develop toxicity such as postoperative, dehydration, hyper-thyroidism, renal disease, or those clients taking diuretics.

You will find LITHIUM on Monitoring Lab Values by the Magic 2s.

DRUG FOR MANIC CLIENT

Levels

Incontinence

Thirst
Thyroid

Hand tremors

Increase fluids

Unsteady

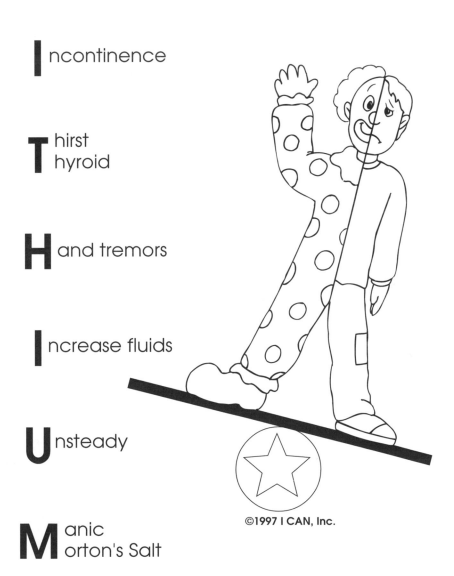

©1997 I CAN, Inc.

Manic
Morton's Salt

SCHIZOPHRENIA

The schizophrenic disorders are **HARD** to deal with. Their behavior is often maladaptive and involves alterations in thinking, moods, feelings, perceptions, communication patterns and interpersonal relationships.

The schizophrenic client has a **HARD** time with relationships and a **HARD** time with the establishment of trust. The word "**HARD**" may help you remember these concepts. It's **HARD** being schizophrenic and it's **HARD** (challenging) providing nursing care.

The nurse said to the person with schizophrenia, "It's time for lunch."

He said, "I'm DEAD, Dead folks don't eat."

She said, "It's time for meds."

He said, "Dead folks don't take meds."

She said, "Time for a bath."

You guessed it. "Dead folks don't bathe either."

How to prove to him that he was not dead? She had a great idea! She asked, "Do dead folks bleed?"

"Of course dead folks don't bleed," he answered.

She went after her needle and syringe and took some blood from his arm, held it up proudly and said, "SEE!"

He said, "I'll be damn, dead folks **do** bleed."

The moral to this story is that they cannot be reasoned with and the nursing care is **HARD**.

SCHIZOPHRENIA

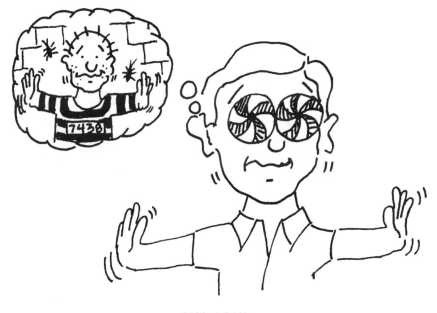

©1994 I CAN

Hallucinations

Affect, ambivalence, autism, associative looseness

Relationship

Delusions

CHARACTERISTICS OF ALCOHOLICS

The general characteristics of an alcoholic have been organized around the "**5 D's**" in order to simplify learning.

D *DENIAL*–The ability to block out or disown the painful thoughts or feelings that he or she has a drinking problem is a major defense mechanism used by the alcoholic.

D *DEPENDENT*–Depends on other people; however, remains resentful of authority. Clients can create codependency in those individuals around them.

D *DEMANDING* –These clients have a low tolerance for frustration.

D *DISSATISFIED*–They tend not to be satisfied with life. There is a tendency toward self-destructive acts including suicide.

D *DOMINEERING*–This behavior is to mask the low self-esteem and poor self-concept.

CHARACTERISTICS OF ALCOHOLICS

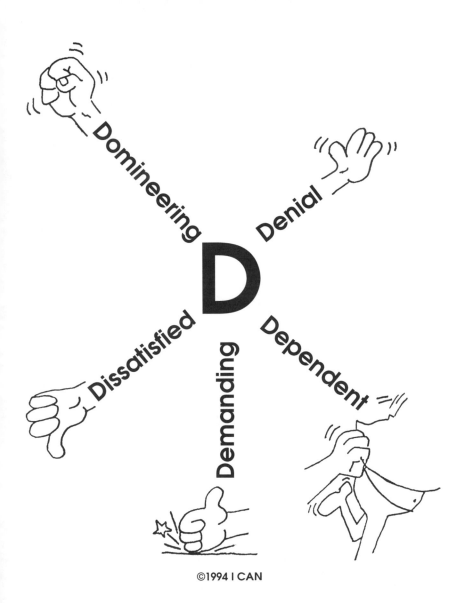

©1994 I CAN

ALCOHOLISM

One of the goals during the long-term rehabilitation is to assist client in identifying alternate coping mechanisms. **"COPES"** is the key in reviewing the priority nursing plans.

C   *COPING MECHANISMS* – Encourage client to develop alternative coping mechanisms other than alcohol to deal with stress. The client must be responsible for sobriety.

O   *ORIENT TO COMMUNITY RESOURCES* – Refer clients to available community resources such as Alcoholics Anonymous (AA), Alanon and Alateen. Abuse of spouses or children often occur while the client is drinking. Notify appropriate protection services for suspected spouse or child abuse.

P   *PLAN* may include antabuse. Antabuse is a drug used by a willing client as a deterrent that will make the client violently ill (flushing, hypotension and nausea and vomiting if he takes it and drinks alcohol). The nurse should always know when the client had the last drink before she administers this drug. *Never administer any medications or substances with alcohol in them (i.e., cough syrup, mouth wash, shaving cream, etc.) while the client is taking antabuse.*

E   *ENCOURAGE DIET* – Vitamin B complex is often used for the alcoholic client with delerium tremens and for the treatment of peripheral neuritis. Alcoholics often have avitaminosis because they drink instead of eat. Folic acid deficiency can lead to obstetrical complications.

S   *SEIZURES* – Delerium Tremens usually occur within 48 hours after cessation of drinking. Picking at the bed covers, tremors of hands, anxiety, nausea, hypertension and nightmares followed by seizures may cause an emergency.

ALCOHOLISM

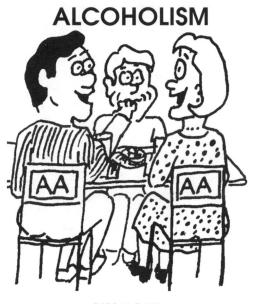

©1994 I CAN

C oping mechanisms

O rient to community resources

P lan may include antabuse

E ncourage vitamin B, folic acid

S eizures

101

DEMENTIA

"The Slow House of Alzheimer's" tells the story of "Poppa" who came to live with his son, but was so confused. The first night Son found Poppa a mile down the road in his pajama shirt and boxer shorts. He had fallen and his leg was bleeding. Poppa was "going to the house" (4 states away). To protect him, Son put a chair in front of his bedroom door, so that when he got up in the middle of the night he would be heard. Poppa would have gone nuts if he had been restrained. Barriers are much safer and more humane.

Son's wife could not wait to take Poppa to the cafeteria dining room so he could choose his own food, but Poppa stood there and stood there. Son's wife had to choose his food because decisions were impossible. The bathroom was a problem. Poppa had used the "out of doors" when he was a boy and his memory had regressed. It was easier to schedule his elimination than to embarrass the neighbors. Unfortunately the schedule was not always accurate and sometimes there were embarrassing wet clothes.

This story is a common one for people with dementia. **"The Slow House of Alzheimer's"** will help you remember the symptoms of **lost** and **wandering, confusion, decision difficulty, incontinence** and **confinement for safety**.

These changes are often progressive and irreversible. The cardinal rule for the geriatric population is do not push too fast (go slowly). It is important to reorient Poppa to the current **reality**. Objects such as clocks and calendars may help. Poppa's self-esteem may benefit through **reminiscing**. He may be able to recall events 10 years ago, but not 10 minutes ago. Poppa needs to be encouraged to remain **independent** as long as possible. Avoid dependency. Develop a plan for activities of daily living and remember **consistency** is important. As Poppa has illustrated, **safety** is very important. Due to sundowners and the increase risk of wandering and falling, **safety** precautions may become a high priority for these clients.

Remember—The difference between dementia (Alzheimer's) and delirium. Dementia is progressive and irreversible. Delirium or acute confusion state can result from sepsis, drug drug interactions, fluid and electrolyte imbalances, etc.

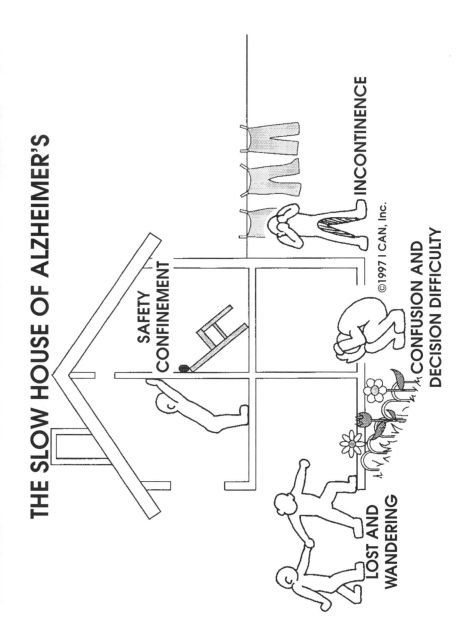

THE SLOW HOUSE OF ALZHEIMER'S

SAFETY CONFINEMENT

INCONTINENCE

CONFUSION AND DECISION DIFFICULTY

LOST AND WANDERING

©1997 I CAN, Inc.

COMBAT

Many people feel they put combat boots on the minute they get up in the morning, but we are referring to the client who is out of control. This may include folks that are real mad, manics, alcoholics, dementias and personality disorders just to name a few. It does not matter what the etiology is; the concept of "**COMBAT**" is still the same.

C   *CONTROL IMMEDIATE SITUATION* – Get their attention. Remove harmful objects. Maintain distance between self and client. Remain neutral.

O   *OUT OF SITUATION* – Remove client from the environment to de-escalate combative behavior.

M   *MAINTAIN CALM* – Do not hurry. Channel the agitated behavior.

B   *BE FIRM AND SET LIMITS* – Be consistent and prevent overt aggression.

A   *AVOID RESTRAINTS* – Use restraints as a last intervention.

T   *TRY CONSEQUENCES* – Positive consequences for positive behavior.

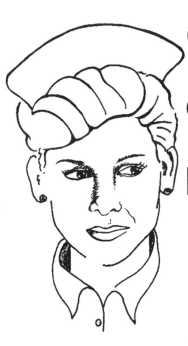

Control immediate

Out of situation

Maintain calm

Be firm/set limits

Avoid restraints

Try consequences

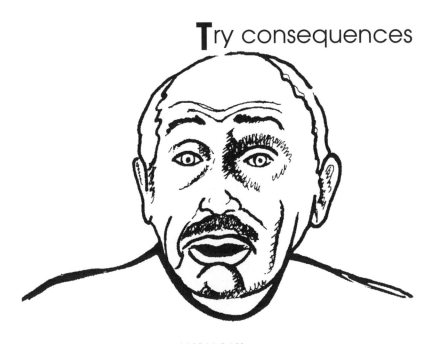

©1994 I CAN

105

VISUAL CHANGES

The images on the next page will help you recall the major eye disorders. **GLAUCOMA** is described by clients as seeing halos around lights. Tunnel vision is another common complaint resulting from an increase in intraocular pressure. Loss of vision can occur. Glaucoma is chronic and a major cause of blindness.

CATARACT is a complete or partial opacity of the lens. This disorder is described as a decrease in visual acuity. Imagine you had on your sunglasses, and we took a paint brush and painted white paint on the outside of your glasses. Could you see out? Of course not. Is it painful? No. That is similar to cataracts.

RETINAL DETACHMENT is described as a sensation of having a veil or curtain over the eye. This disorder is sudden in onset. Some clients may experience an area of blank vision. Retinal detachment occurs from a separation of the two layers of the retina. When separation occurs, vitreous humor seeps between the layers and detachment of the retina from the choroid occurs.

MACULAR DEGENERATION is described as a blind spot in the center of the field of vision. Peripheral vision is retained but client is unable to read, drive, etc. There is no cure at this time.

VISUAL CHANGES

Glaucoma

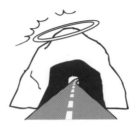 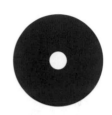

Halo tunnel

Cataracts

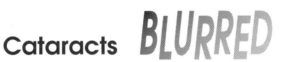 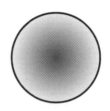

Blurred

Retinal detachment

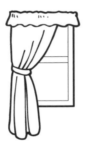 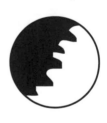

Curtain

Macular degeneration

BLACK SP🖤T

Black spot

MYDRIATICS

The word mydriatics has a **D** for *dilate* and an **A** for *atropine*. When you think about this, it will help you remember that **MYDRIATICS** dilate the eye for eye exams and eye surgery. Atropine, epinephrine, cyclogyl and mydriacyl are commonly used mydriatics. Would we want people with glaucoma to receive atropine? Not usually.

DILATE EYES:
EYE EXAM

MYDRIATICS

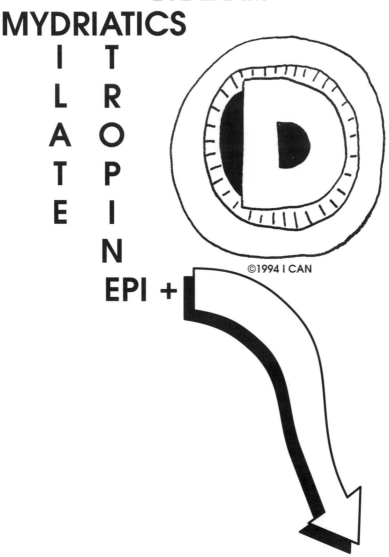

D I L A T E

T R O P I N

EPI +

©1994 I CAN

CyclogYL
MYDRIAcYL

MIOTICS

Miotics are given to people who have an elevated pressure in the eye due to glaucoma. The word miotics has a **C** in it for *constrict*. As a result of the constriction from these drugs, there is an increased flow of the aqueous humor. Interestingly enough, many of the miotic eye drops contain the word **CAR**. **CARpine**, **CARbachol**, and **piloCARpine** are all miotics.

Notice the tag on our friend's car. He "*KANT C*" well due to his tunnel vision. Clients with primary open-angle glaucoma experience a gradual loss of peripheral vision which is described as "tunnel vision." *Isn't that EASY?*

CONSTRICT EYES:
GLAUCOMA

MIOTICS

C
O
N
S
T
R
I
C
T

NO ATROPINE!!

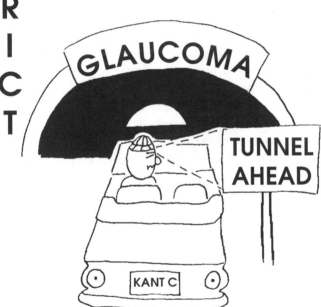

GLAUCOMA

TUNNEL
AHEAD

KANT C

©1994 I CAN

CARpine
CARbachol
pilo**CAR**

EAR DROPS

Aren't these guys great! They have been "mascots" on our marketing materials since 1991. They epitomize Accelerated Learning.

The ear canal changes as we grow. To be sure that ear drops can get down into the ear, we need to remember how to hold the ear when we're putting in those drops. Notice the word *adult* has a **U** in it for **UP**. Hold the adult ear **UP** and back. Notice that the word *child* ends in a **D**. Hold the child's ear **DOWN** and back.

WHEN INSTALLING EAR DROPS REMEMBER THAT THE EAR IS

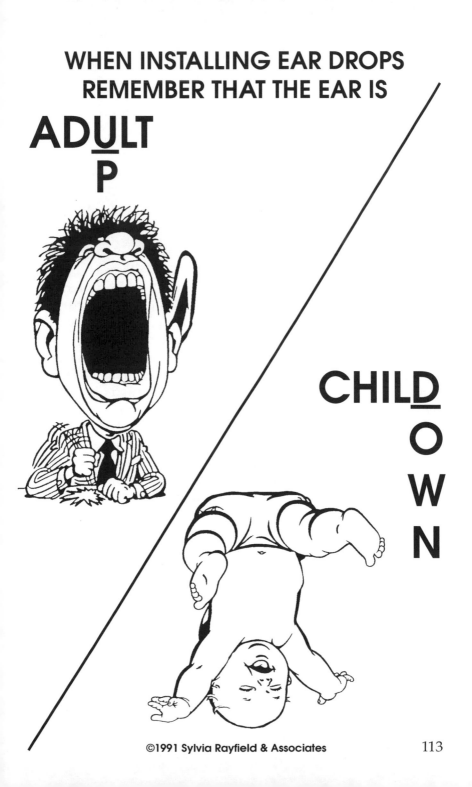

SIADH

Soggy Sid has SIADH (syndrome of inappropriate antidiuretic hormone), a condition that continually releases the antidiuretic hormone (ADH). With increased ADH, the body retains water and gets so Soggy that water intoxication may occur.

Sid's cap is hiding his bandaged head from a head injury, which is a major risk factor for SIADH. Due to his cerebral edema, he is prone to seizures. Notice his limbs are small. There is no obvious edema, yet he has gained weight in his body. The intake and output record will document low urinary output because he's keeping it all on board. The urine specific gravity will be high. The serum sodium will be decreased (dilutional). Limit Soggy Sid's fluid intake. He may be given diuretics to assist with fluid excretion, especially if he has respiratory or cardiac problems. Keep Soggy Sid's bed flat or only slightly elevated. This position of his head will decrease the secretion of ADH. Keep the neuro checks going. Soggy Sid is in serious condition!

SOGGY SID

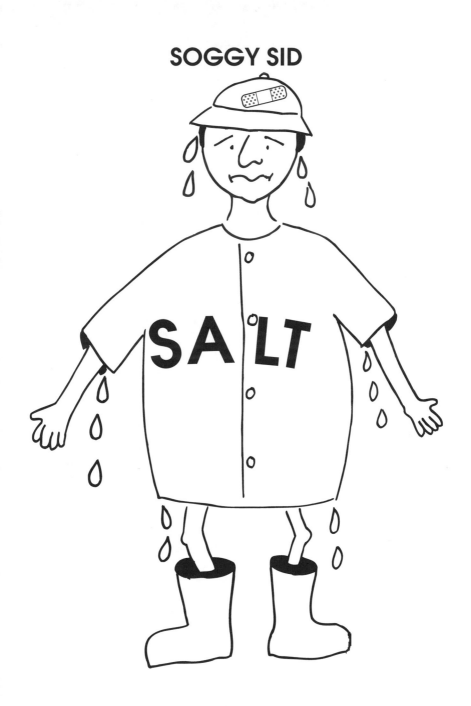

HYPERTHYROIDISM

GO GETTER GERTRUDE will help you remember the major symptoms of hyperthyroidism. Her last name, of course, is Graves. Graves' disease is the result of hyperthyroidism. One look at this visually stunning creature, and you can see how thin she is and how her eyes "bug out" (exophthalmus). Everything is running except her menstrual periods. Her HEART is running fast (increased pulse), her BLOOD PRESSURE is running UP, and her basal metabolic rate (BMR) is running, therefore the metabolism of drugs will be faster. She can eat a whole chocolate cake without ever gaining an ounce. She is running so much that she is cleaning out closets that don't need cleaning at 3:00 in the morning. Notice she is wearing short sleeves and pants because it takes a lot of energy to run, and she is hot all the time. While planning her nursing care, lower the room temperature and get rid of all those excess blankets. A quiet room will be great! Well-balanced meals (high in calories and vitamins) is a must. Due to the eye changes, protect cornea from drying. GO GETTER'S diagnostic tests would reveal an increase in the following reports: T3 and T4, protein bound iodine (PBI), BMR, and uptake of I 131. (Refer to **Hypothyroidism.**)

GO GETTER GERTRUDE

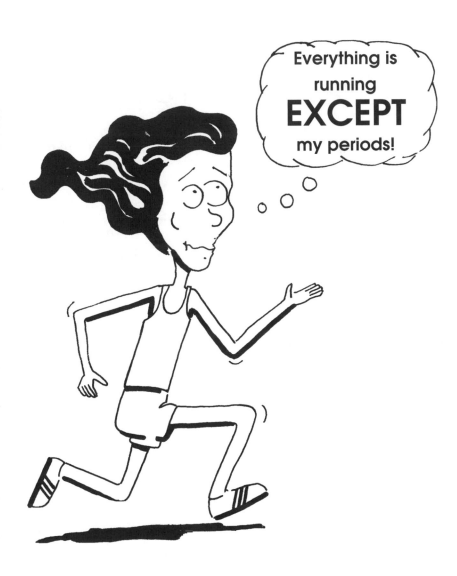

THYROIDECTOMY

The **BOW TIE** is around his neck because the hyperactive thyroid gland has been removed. Post-op can be a crucial period for these folks because they may *BLEED*. Often the blood collects behind the neck, being pulled by gravity if he is lying on his back. Place him in semi-Fowler's position to avoid tension on the suture line. Observe the *AIRWAY* due to potential swelling from being traumatized during surgery. Vocal chords may be swollen. Assess frequently for noisy breathing and increased restlessness. Evaluate *VOCAL* changes; increasing hoarseness may be indicative of laryngeal edema. If these people get into trouble they can lose their airway fast. It's advisable to have a *TRACHEOTOMY SET* available to open an emergency airway. The *INCISION* needs to be observed for swelling which can occlude the airway. Watch for normal wound healing. We don't want an infection. Evaluate calcium levels; parathyroids may have been damaged or accidentally removed. Since calcium potentiates the movement of electrolytes across the cell membrane and electrolyte balance is imperative for the heart cells to work, low levels could create an *EMERGENCY*. Have calcium gluconate available!

POST-OP THYROIDECTOMY

Bleeding

Open airway

Whisper

Trache set

Incision

Emergency

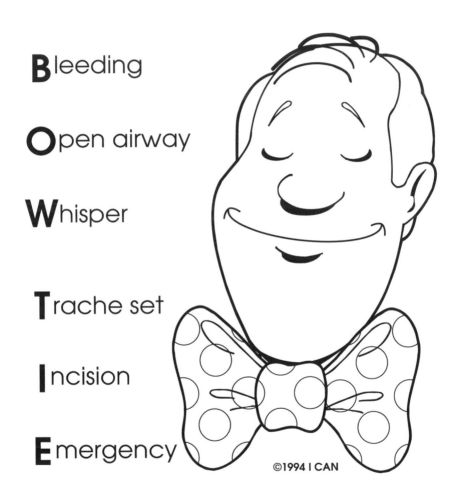

©1994 I CAN

HYPOTHYROIDISM

This vision of loveliness is **MORBID MATILDA**. Her last name, as you've probably guessed, is Myxedema (Hypothyroid). She has a slow deterioration of the thyroid function. It occurs mostly in older adults and five times more frequently in women than in men.

As you can see, Matilda has the family "bug-eyes" and she has no menstrual period like her sister Gertrude, but that's where the resemblance ends. (Refer to **Hyperthyroidism**.) Matilda is not thin. In fact, she can look at a piece of chocolate cake and gain weight. She had rather sleep at 3:00 in the morning than clean closets. She may also be sleeping at 3:00 in the afternoon because of her lack of energy. Her long pants and putting her hands in her pocket will keep her warm. Increasing the room temperature may be necessary.

Matilda will be placed on lifelong thyroid replacement, and will be on a low-calorie, low cholesterol diet to help with her weight loss. Morbid Matilda does not like these changes. She is definitely not a very happy camper!

MORBID MATILDA

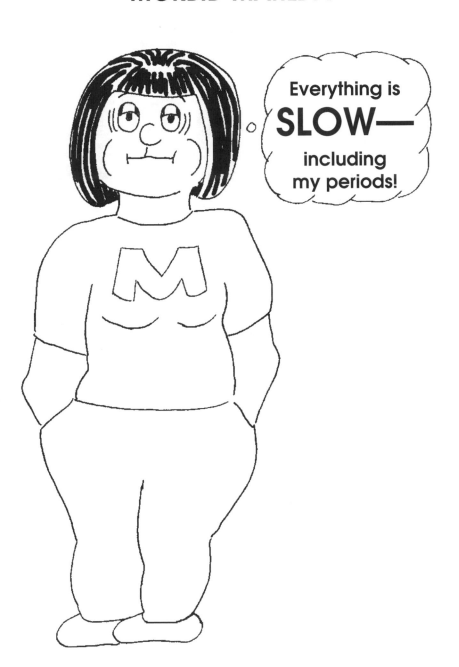

DIABETES MELLITUS

FIDO, the diabetic dog, is exhibiting all of the signs and symptoms of hyperglycemia. Sugar is floating around in his blood stream because there is no insulin to take the sugar into the cells.

Since the cells are starving for lack of sugar, Fido is dreaming of food. He has a huge appetite. His food bowl in front of him remains empty because he keeps trying to feed those starving cells (POLYPHAGIA). The high sugar content in his blood is pulling fluid from the cells which makes him very thirsty (POLYDIPSIA). Since his kidneys are compensating by dumping extra fluid and sugar out onto the street (POLY-URIA), he has totally wet down the fire hydrant. Look at Fido's pants! They don't fit any more. The sugar and the fluid that he has taken in have not gone into his cells, since there is no insulin to assist in crossing over into the cell. As a result, poor Fido has LOST WEIGHT. What medication would you plan to have available? Insulin of course. (Refer to **Hypoglycemia.**)

WHAT'S WRONG WITH FIDO?

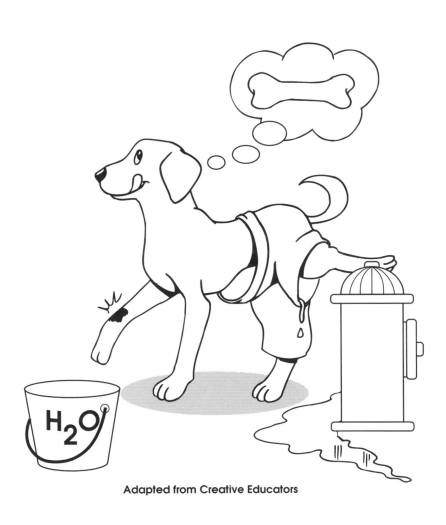

Adapted from Creative Educators

INSULIN

Do you have difficulty remembering the onset, peak, and duration of the various types of insulin? Let us help simplify this for you, so it will be easy!! In your mind it will be helpful to categorize the rapid, intermediate, and long acting insulin. The onset of the rapid acting insulin is 30 - 60 minutes. If you can recall this time frame being real fast, then you will be able to remember the other insulin. For the intermediate insulin, multiply 60 x 2 and the onset is 60 - 120 minutes. For the long acting insulin, multiply 120 x 2 and the onset is 240 min. (4 hrs.) - 480 min. (8 hrs.).

As you can see on caps on the next page, the peak has a general progression. Humalog and Regular start with a peak of 3 hours progressing by 2 hours for a peak action for the semilente being 5 - 7 hrs. Add 1 - 5 hrs. to the 7 hrs. for the NPH peak action being 8 - 12 hrs. As you can see the lente peak went up by 3 hrs. for the range peak being 7 - 15 hrs. and the ultralente increased by 5 from the 15 hr. peak action of the lente. These will assist you in remembering the average peak action for your examination.

The duration of Humalog is 5 hrs. The remainder of the times are in increments of 6. The regular insulin's duration is 6 hrs. Multiply that by 2 and the semilente is 12 - 16 hrs. Multiply 12 by 2 and the NPH and Lente insulin have a duration of 24 hrs. The Ultralente insulin has the longest duration of 36 hrs. See HYPOGLYCEMIA for insulin reaction.

Remember–Regular insulin is the only insulin which may be given IV.

PEAK TIMES FOR INSULIN

LONG
4 HOURS (240 MINUTES)

PEAK 16–20 hrs
DURATION 36

ULTRALENTE

INTERMEDIATE
ONSET 60–120 MINUTES

PEAK 7–15 hrs
DURATION 24

LENTE

PEAK 8–12 hrs
DURATION 24

NPH

©1997 I CAN, Inc.

SHORT
ONSET 30–60 MINUTES

PEAK 5–7 hrs
DURATION 12–16

SEMILENTE

PEAK 3 hrs
DURATION 6

REGULAR

PEAK 3 hrs
DURATION 5

HUMALOG

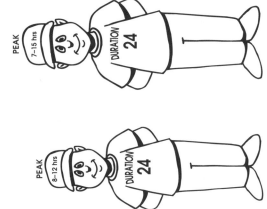

125

HYPOGLYCEMIA

People taking insulin may have hypoglycemic reactions. This is a fact. Some diabetics have them everyday; others rarely have this problem. Teach them the symptoms, so they recognize their situation. Some of the signs and symptoms to observe are they may get suddenly **TIRED** and run out of steam. *TACHYCARDIA* (rapid pulse) occurs as a warning. *TREMORS* or nervousness are other warning signs. They often become *IRRITABLE* and *RESTLESS*. They may mow anyone down in the coke line to get some food due to *EXCESSIVE HUNGER*. They know if they don't, they may be out! *DIA-PHORESIS* is common, and is an excellent guideline for determining if the client is asleep versus having a hypoglycemic reaction. If the client is unconscious, administer glucagon IV. Encourage them to eat carbohydrates or drink milk if they are awake.

*If ever in doubt of a diagnosis of hypoglycemia versus hyperglycemia, give carbohydrates–severe hypoglycemia can result in permanent brain damage.

Remember this jingle to help recall the differences:

COLD AND CLAMMY MEANS YOU NEED SOME CANDY
HOT AND DRY MEANS YOUR SUGAR IS HIGH.

Jingle reprinted with permission, NEC, Dallas, Texas

SYMPTOMS OF HYPOGLYCEMIA

Tremors
Tachycardia

Irritability

Restless

Excessive hunger

Diaphoresis
Depression

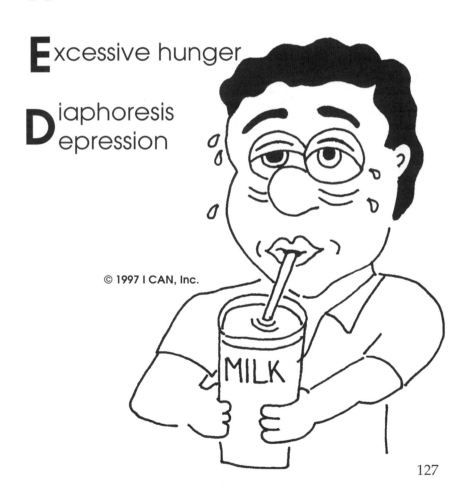

© 1997 I CAN, Inc.

127

CUSHING'S SYNDROME

One look at **CUSHY CARL** and you see his problem. He has an overproduction of hormones from the adrenal cortex. As you see, he's holding a "twinkie." These people may have a HIGH BLOOD SUGAR. The bag of chips he is holding indicates his INCREASE in SODIUM resulting in fluid retention. Increase in volume naturally will ELEVATE the BLOOD PRESSURE. Watch that POTASSIUM level, it will have a tendency to DECREASE and we certainly do not want his heart doing any strange dances (arrhythmias). Cushy's fat face also let's us know he's holding fluids. His "buffalo hump" probably scares him enough that his blood pressure goes up even higher. The sore on his leg won't heal because of his high blood sugar. (Would we want to protect him from INFECTION? You bet!)

Put 2 and 2 together. Would we want to give a diabetic steroids? Not if we can help it. Sometimes there are no options, so if this is the case, monitor the blood sugar. Now we know that cortisone (steroids) will increase the blood sugar even higher, increase edema, and increase the risk for infection. With all of this going on, Cushy will indeed need some assistance with his emotional state.

We know we would! What about you?

CUSHY CARL

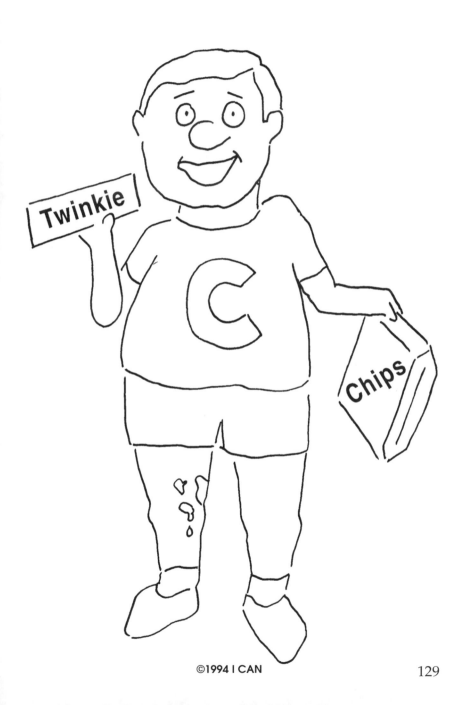

ADDISON'S DISEASE

ANEMIC ADAM, whose last name is Addison, is Cushy Carl's half brother.(Refer to **Cushing's Syndrome**.) The whole family thinks they have opposite characteristics. Adam has a disorder which is caused by a decrease in secretion of the adrenal cortex hormone.

Adam craves salt since he doesn't have enough. That is the reason he is out in the field at the salt lick. Hyponatremia has a tendency to cause low blood pressure. In addition, his potassium may be increased. He has hypoglycemia and complains of being tired and weak much of the time. This weakness is a cardinal complaint and usually is more severe in times of stress. Occasionally, Adam stays in bed. After his anorexia, nausea, vomiting and diarrhea, he is dehydrated and has a serious loss in weight. After all of this, who wouldn't be tired and weak? His skin has turned bronze, and it is not due to too much sun. This is caused by increased levels of melanocyte stimulating hormone (MSH). To prevent addisonian crisis, corticosteroids will have to be replaced.

ANEMIC ADAM

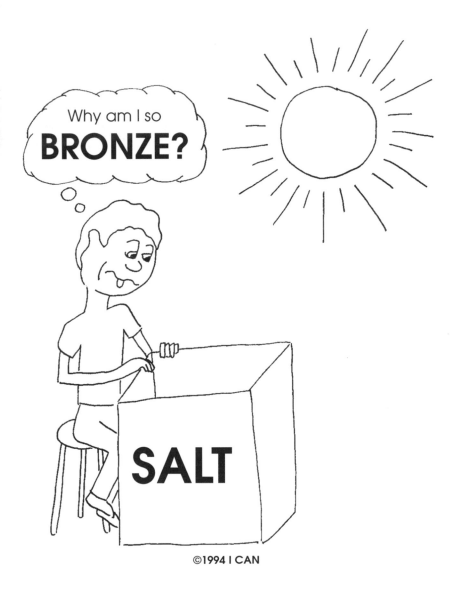

SICKLE CELL ANEMIA

Sickle cell anemia is characterized by the sickling effect of erythrocytes (red blood cells)–results in increased blood viscosity and increased red cell destruction. Increased viscosity eventually precipitates ischemia and tissue necrosis due to capillary stasis and thrombosis. The image for this condition is a rabbit on a bicycle (**BiSICKLE**). How do rabbits get around? Of course we know they "**HOP**" "**HOP**"!

H **HYDRATION**–Viscosity may be decreased with adequate IV fluids. Monitor IV fluids and encourage fluid intake. Sluggish circulation may cause an electrolyte imbalance. Be aware of fluid and electrolyte imbalances caused by temperature elevations, vomiting and diarrhea, etc.

O *OXYGEN*–Administer oxygen. Adequate oxygen helps prevent sickling from occurring. Avoid fatigue, traveling to high altitude areas, aircraft travel or participating in a strenuous activity.

P *PAIN MEDICINE*–Due to their extreme discomfort, analgesics will be given.

S *SUPPORT*–Support the parents by encouraging genetic counseling. Child may be supported by providing normal developmental activities.

SICKLE CELL ANEMIA

Hydrate

Oxygen

Pain medicine

Support

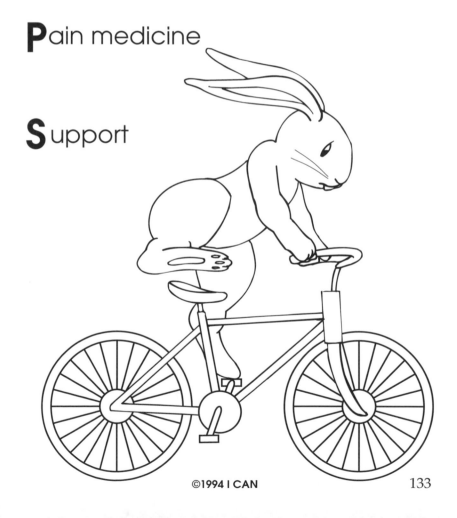

BLOOD TRANSFUSION REACTIONS

With both allergic and hemolytic reactions, the nursing intervention is the same. **STOP** the transfusion immediately! The reactions for both allergic and hemolytic have been outlined on the next page.

After stopping the transfusion, change the IV tubing; do not allow blood in the tubing to infuse into the client. Blood samples may be drawn by the lab. If client has a history of allergic reaction, Benadryl may be given prior to starting the infusion.

Before, during, or after the transfusion, DO NOT use D5W; it causes the blood to hemolyze then precipitate. **Normal Saline** is the crystalloid of choice. Always use a blood administration set with a filter; DO NOT use straight IV tubing. Start the infusion at approximately 20 drops per minute (100 cc per hour) for about 15 to 20 minutes; remain with the client during this time. If a reaction occurs, it is most likely to occur within the first 15 minutes. During the transfusion, continue to monitor for circulatory overload or transfusion reaction. One unit of blood should not hang longer than 4 hours.

Remember–The majority of major adverse transfusion reactions are due to improper identification of the blood product and the client!

BLOOD TRANSFUSION REACTIONS

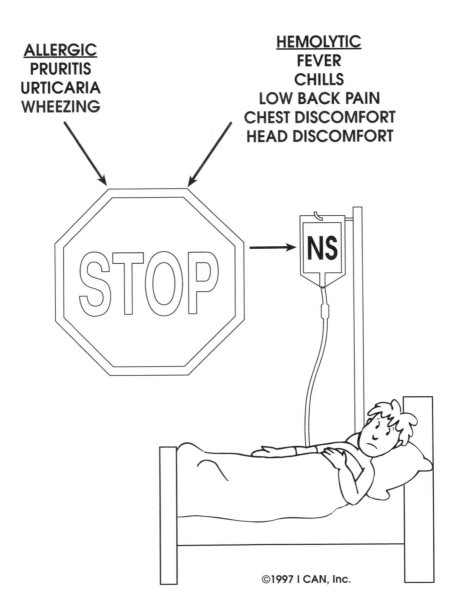

ALLERGIC
PRURITIS
URTICARIA
WHEEZING

HEMOLYTIC
FEVER
CHILLS
LOW BACK PAIN
CHEST DISCOMFORT
HEAD DISCOMFORT

©1997 I CAN, Inc.

SIDE EFFECTS OF CHEMOTHERAPY

BARRY **BARFS** is pretty miserable taking those chemotherapeutic drugs! Those drugs cause *BONE MARROW DEPRESSION* resulting in a decrease in the platelet count. Observe Barry for bruising or bleeding. His gums are particularly vulnerable to bleeding. Barry may want to use an electric razor and a soft-bristle toothbrush. Bone marrow depression can also cause leukopenia. If we don't have enough white blood cells, we must assess for elevated temperature and possible infection. Barry should be isolated from communicable diseases, especially chicken pox. Anemia is also a common side effect because bone marrow depression suppresses red cell formation. Maintain adequate rest. Organize activities to avoid fatigue. Notice Barry only has three twigs in the middle of his bald head. The drugs have caused *ALOPECIA. RETCHING* (nausea and vomiting) makes it hard to maintain fluid and electrolyte balance. Small feedings with increased fluids will help! Meticulous oral hygiene and anesthetic mouth wash may help the *STOMATITIS*.

When Barry is this sick, it is natural to be *FEARFUL* and *ANXIOUS*. We can help by being compassionate and allowing him to verbalize his fears and concerns. Your support is very important! HUMANIZE YOUR CARE!

SIDE EFFECTS OF CHEMOTHERAPY

Bone marrow depression

Alopecia

Retching—nausea/vomiting

Fear and anxiety

Stomatitis

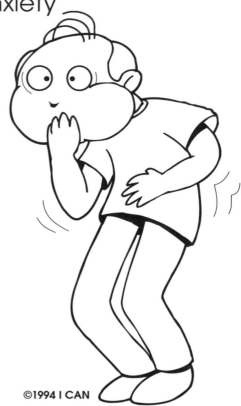

©1994 I CAN

CYANOTIC HEART DEFECTS

Some folks have a hard time remembering which of those congenital heart defects are cyanotic versus which are acyanotic.

NO PROBLEM, just remember all congenital heart defects that begin with the letter "T" are cyanotic defects. Color the "T" on the next page blue to help you remember this easy concept.

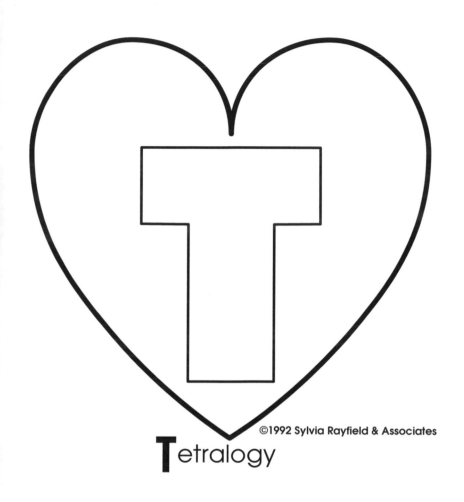

Tetralogy

Truncus

Transposition

Tricuspid

TETRALOGY OF FALLOT

Tetralogy of Fallot is often referred to as that complicated congenital heart defect that causes children to "squat" or "**DROP**" to the floor. When they get tired or out of breath, this position will decrease the amount of venous return to the heart. **DROP** will assist you in reviewing the four physiological defects with the heart in Tetralogy of Fallot.

D Displaced aorta which allows unoxygenated blood into the oxygenated system causing cyanosis (overriding aorta).

R Right Ventricle hypertrophies due to working so hard pumping against pressure. The more the heart muscle works the bigger it gets.

O Opening in the septum is a "hole" that allows shunting of unoxygenated blood to mix with oxygenated blood (ventricular septal defect).

P Pulmonary valve partially closes making the right ventricle work, thus causing the right ventricle to hypertrophy.

These children are often small, tired, delicate and need surgery before leading a better quality of life. Teach parents to pace the child's activities, provide good nutrition to build strength and to renew themselves. Due to the challenges of these children, the parents need emotional support!

TETRALOGY OF FALLOT

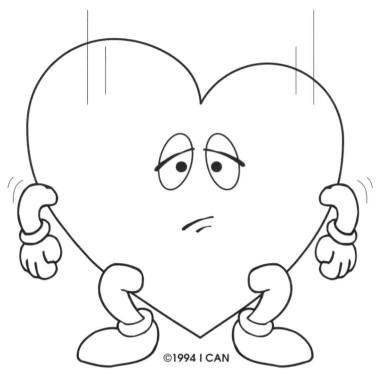

©1994 I CAN

Displaced aorta

Right ventricle hypertrophy

Opening in septum

Pulmonary valve stenosis

141

HEARTS

This is to assist with remembering the nursing evaluation for an infant who has a serious defect requiring home care prior to corrective surgery. Think of a **HEART** since this is the location of surgery.

H   *HEART MURMUR* – A murmur will be assessed especially with ventricular septal defects (VSD), atrial septal defects (ASD), and patent ductus arteriosus (PDA).

E   *EVALUATE WEIGHT GAIN* – Due to their intolerance to suck well, they will have a slow weight gain. Some of these infants will be fed via a feeding tube because of their weakness.

A   *ACTIVITY INTOLERANCE* – The infant fatigues easily. Conserve oxygen by anticipating their needs, so they won't cry.

R   *RESPIRATORY INFECTIONS* – Due to pooling of blood in the pulmonary region, these infants have an increased frequency in respiratory infections.

T   *TACHYCARDIA* – An elevation in the resting heart and respiratory rate are signs of hypoxia. Assess these changes carefully! They will give you a lot of information.

S   *SUPPORT* – Allow family to grieve over loss of perfect infant. Foster early parent-infant attachment; encourage touching, holding and loving.

ASSESSMENTS FOR CONGENITAL HEART DISEASE

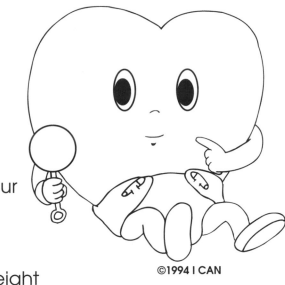

©1994 I CAN

Heart murmur

Evaluate weight

Activity intolerance

Respiratory infections

Tachycardia & Tachypnea

Support

143

HYPERTENSION

Catapres, a commonly used antihypertensive, is the name of our image to review RISK FACTORS. Just look at this gorgeous black woman. (Studies show that women of color have hypertension more often than other races.) See letters on the next page as you read below.

C People with hypertension may have small capillary hemorrhages in their eyes, blurred vision, and headaches.

A Nose bleeds could occur causing anxiety which leads to a further blood pressure increase.

T Carotid endarterectomies may be performed to prevent or relieve symptoms of a CVA caused from atherosclerosis of arteries in the throat.

A Her wide girth, obesity and hypertension go hand in hand.

P Pheochromocytoma and adrenal tumors can cause hypertension.

R Notice the feet; diabetics are known to have hypertension. Thickened toe nails and foot ulcers may result in gangrene.

E E stands for "Essential" hypertension (unknown cause). Early high blood pressure may have few symptoms.

S Sexual dysfunction may occur as a result from the medicines.

HEALTH PROMOTION IS A MUST!

CATAPRES

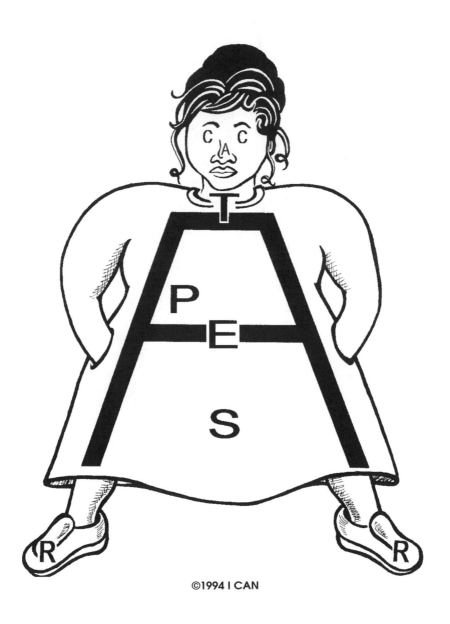

©1994 I CAN

HYPERTENSIVE MEDICATIONS

C *COMPLIANCE* – Clients without symptoms may not take meds, especially if meds cause more symptoms than the high blood pressure.

A *ACE INHIBITORS* (angiotensin converting enzymes, ACE) are a group of drugs which lower the blood pressure (ie., capoten and vasotec). Monitor the blood pressure, especially on the first dose which may cause hypotension. Evaluate blood pressure if on diuretics.

T *THIAZIDES* such as Esidrix, Enduron, and Hygroton decrease the blood volume, by increasing the urinary output like crazy! Teach client to take these meds in the morning, otherwise they will be up half the night going to the bathroom.

A *ALDACTONE* and Lasix are other drugs commonly used to treat hypertension: watch the urinary output go *up, up, up*.

P *PRESSURE*– The national definition of hypertension is 140/90.

R *RISK* factors should be addressed through education.

E *ELECTROLYTES* , especially K^+, gets dumped down the toilet when diuretics are taken.

S *SEXUAL* function may be diminished.

CATAPRES II

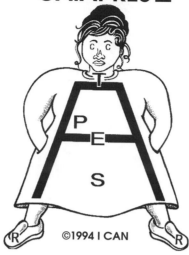

©1994 I CAN

Compliance

Ace inhibitors

Thiazides

Aldactone

Pressure

Risk factors

Electrolytes

Sexually impotent

147

ACE INHIBITORS

What is an ACE Inhibitor?

It lowers blood pressure by stopping the angiotensin converting enzyme (ACE) in the lung, which reduces the vasoconstrictor, angiotensin II. In other words, when you are playing cards, you may block the aces so your opponent will not win. This indeed will lower your blood pressure.

How do I remember all of these medications?

It's actually insanely easy!!! Remember they are pills and if you put an r after the p, you have a pril; these medications all end in **pril**.

> Capto**pril**
> Enala**pril**
> Lisino**pril**
> Fosino**pril**
> Rami**pril**
> Benzae**pril**

What do I need to evaluate?

1. Blood pressure - Since these medications reduce vasoconstriction, the pressure may go down too low. Observe for dizziness and/or tachycardia.

2. Some undesirable effects include an annoying dry cough, angioedema of the face, lips, tongue, and pharynx. Uncommon side effects include rash and taste disturbances.

3. Monitor for hyponatremia and hyperkalemia.

4. With Captopril, agranulocytosis or neutropenia may occur (ask about sore throats).

ACE INHIBITORS

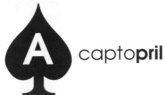 capto**pril**

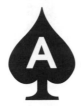 enala**pril**

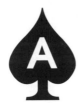 lisino**pril**

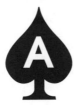 fosino**pril**

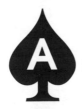 rami**pril**

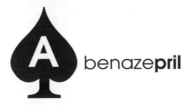 benaze**pril**

149

BETA BLOCKERS

Beta Blockers are a group of drugs that can be remembered using the acronym BETA. People taking these drugs may need TLC (tender loving care).

B *BROCHOSPASM* (so we don't want to give them to people with asthma or brochoconstrictive disease!)

E *ELICITS A DECREASE IN CARDIAC OUTPUT AND CONTRACTILITY.*

T *TREATS HYPERTENSION.*

A *AV CONDUCTION DECREASES* (short for treats arrhythmias, especially fast ones by decreasing the heart rate and cardiac output!)

REMEMBER–STOP BETA BLOCKERS WITH BRONCHOCONSTRICTIVE DISEASE

T *TENORMIN* (atenolol) used for hypertension and angina (watch for renal impairment as this drug is renally excreted).

L *LOPRESSOR* (metoptolol) used for hypertension and angina (contraindicated in sinus bradycardia, 2nd or 3rd degree block, metabolized in liver and NOT renally excreted).

C *CORGARD* (nadolol) used for hypertension and angina (renally excreted, contraindicated in bronchial asthma, sinus bradycardia or 2nd or 3rd degree heart block).

NOTICE ALL THE GENERIC NAMES END IN "LOL"!

ROAD BLOCKS TO BETA BLOCKERS

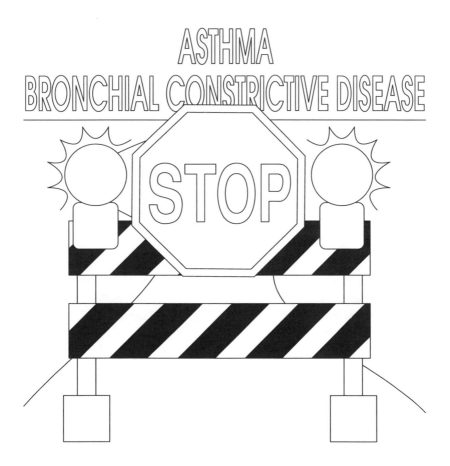

©1997 I CAN, Inc.

CALCIUM CHANNEL BLOCKERS

This group of medications are often called "Don't Give a Shit Pills" by the clients who take them because that's exactly how they feel. Their blood pressure is lowered (calcium influx blocked), pulse is decreased, and if they move too quickly they get dizzy. They are much happier being a couch potato and taking life easy. A few examples of the calcium channel blockers include **Ca**rdizem, **Ca**rdene, Pro**ca**rdia, and **Ca**lan. Each of these common Calcium Channel Blockers have a **Ca** in them which makes it easy to remember! These medications should be administered with meals and milk. Some general undesirable effects of these medications include **constipation, bradycardia, peripheral edema, hypotension, dizziness, heart blocks, and worsening of CHF.**

*Remember–Calcium Channel blockers should **not** be given in clients who are in **congestive heart failure** or **cardiogenic shock** because they can decrease the heart rate too much.*

CALCIUM CHANNEL BLOCKERS

"DON'T GIVE A SHIT PILLS"

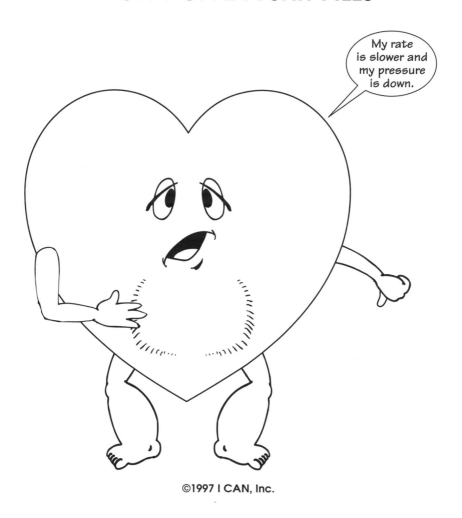

©1997 I CAN, Inc.

LOOP DIURETICS

Lou La Bell has been given a loop diuretic such as Lasix or Ethacrynate Sodium and is very **dizzy**. Her blood pressure has decreased too much after her excessive peeing. You would also feel as if you were spinning in a tube over the falls if you lost this much urine (volume). It may be very useful to teach her to get up slowly so she won't fall.

The life guard must blow his whistle in order to get her some assistance. She feels that the **ringing** in her ears just won't go away. **Dizziness** and **ringing** in the ears are major adverse reactions from loop diuretics.

A few other adverse reactions include: **hypokalemia, hypocalcemia (tetany), hyperglycemia, and hyperuricemia.** While **aplastic anemia and agranulocytosis** may occur, they are RARE!

Remember—Keep a close watch on blood pressure, potassium and calcium levels. Teach foods high in potassium and calcium. See ABC Fruit and Veggie Plate. Potassium supplements may be necessary.

LOU LA BELL

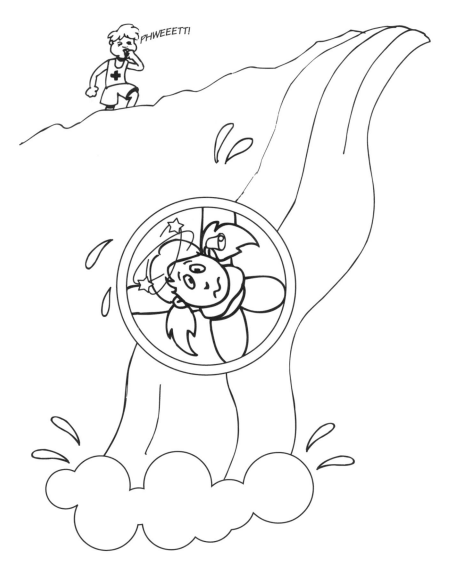

ATRIAL DYSRHYTHMIAS

Atrial actions include Atrial Fibrillation and Atrial Flutter. **DIGITALIS** (Dig) is the drug commonly given to increase cardiac output resulting in a slower heart rate. Digitalis can be both a curse and a cure. Yes, it does convert dysrhythmias back to a normal sinus rhythm, but it can also cause "bradys and blocks" (bradycardia and heart blocks). A drug with a similar conversion effect is *QUINIDINE*.

If these or other drugs won't work, ELECTIVE CARDIOVERSION (*LIE EM DOWN and SHOCK EM*) may become necessary. Push the synchronizer button on the defibrillator prior to cardioversion. The cardioversion may be painful due to the electric current going through the chest, therefore meds such as valium I.V. may be given at the time of cardioversion (shock).

*Be prepared for the cardioversion to convert the rhythm to ventricular tachycardia or ventricular fibrillation. As our mothers always told us, too much of a good thing can be bad for us. Sometimes "stuff just happens"!

ATRIAL ACTIONS

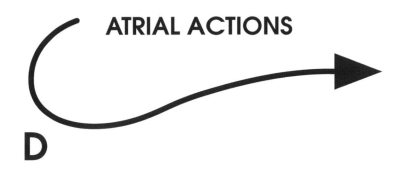

D

Qu**I**nidine

G

I

T

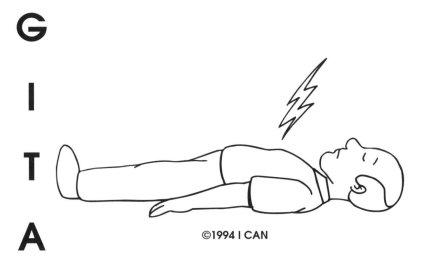

©1994 I CAN

A

Lie 'em and shock 'em

I

S

HEART BLOCKS

A post graduate course in dysrhythmias will certainly provide more detailed information. The bottom line in heart blocks, whether it is 1st, 2nd, or 3rd degree, is when the **PACEMAKER** in the heart (SA node) is delayed or dysfunctional. Drugs commonly used to treat this problem include **ATROPINE, EPINEPHRINE**, and **ISUPREL**. Atropine blocks the vagus nerve impulses on the SA node causing an increased heart rate. Epinephrine will increase bradycardia and increase myocardial contractility. Isuprel increases the ventricular rate and enhances cardiac conduction. This jingle will help in recalling **ISUPREL**:

ISUPREL IS A SOUTHERN BELLE.
SHE MAKES HEADS TURN AND HEART RATES GO UP!

If these drugs fail and a third degree or complete block persists, a mechanical temporary or permanent artificial pacemaker may be inserted by the physician.

*If a pacemaker is inserted, teach client how to monitor their pulse which is an indicator of pacemaker function. Teach symptoms of pacemaker dysfunction and pertinent detail regarding "power" failure in permanent pacemakers. Provide a safe environment by eliminating all possible electrical hazards. Instruct these clients to wear medical identification.

HEART BLOCKS

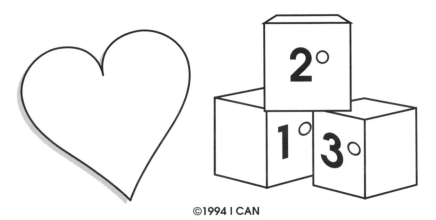

©1994 I CAN

PACEMAKER

T   P

R   ISUPREL

O

P

I

N

E

VENTRICULAR FIBRILLATION

A typical page out of a course manual for ACLS (Acute Cardiac Life Support) would reflect approximately 20 steps of interventions with this dysrhythmia. This material presently is not being taught by many nursing schools, as it is often considered post-graduate information.

We've included parts of it, however, to give you 2 major ideas.

1. A general idea of what to expect during a cardiac arrest.
2. The material that often looks the most difficult can be reduced to INSANELY EASY.

Epinephrine, Lidocaine and Bretylium are several of the drugs used in ventricular fibrillation.

Defibrillate, Defibrillate, Defibrillate,
Epinephrine, Defibrillate,
Lidocaine, Defibrillate,
Bretylium, Defibrillate,
Bretylium, Defibrillate,
Lidocaine, Defibrillate

Refer to next page for an easy way to remember these steps!

Defibrillate = Shock
Epinephrine = Everybody
Lidocaine = Little
Bretylium = Big

Shock Shock Shock
EVERYBODY SHOCK

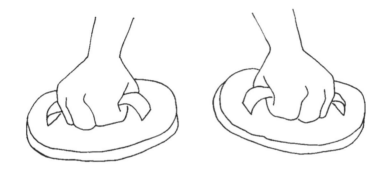

Little shock - BIG SHOCK
BIG SHOCK - Little shock

ACID-BASE

Draw a line down the middle of the right page. At the top of the left column put the numbers 7.35. At the top of the right column put 7.45. The normal blood pH should stay between these numbers. A pH below 7.35 indicates acidosis. A pH above 7.45 indicates alkalosis. Under 7.35 write CO_2 (body turns carbon dioxide to carbonic acid). Under 7.45 write HCO_3. Under HCO_3 write HCO_3 again and again. If we had enough paper we would write HCO_3 20 times because normal ratio of HCO_3 to pCO_2 is 20:1. The objective is to keep the pH between 7.35 and 7.45 which is done with buffer systems.

COLOR the van red. The red van represents the blood buffer system. Imagine the van driving through the arteries and veins of your body. When the pH gets below 7.35 (acidosis) the back van door opens, out jumps 20 little bicarbs, neutralizes the acid and gets back in the van to drive off! If the ph gets above 7.45 (alkalosis) the front van door opens, big powerful CO_2 jumps out, neutralizes and gets back in to drive off. This blood buffer is the first buffer system to respond to pH variations. The lungs follow by adjusting the respirations to regulate the CO_2. The third buffer system that helps maintain the pH are the kidneys.

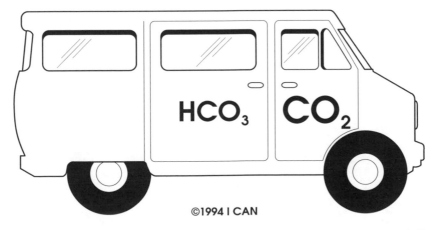

©1994 I CAN

ACID-BASE STATUS

To determine acid-base status (respiratory or metabolic), picture yourself in Rome. You are on a playground with Phonetia (pH), Carbo (HCO_3), and Paco (pCO_2).

Phonetia and Paco hop on the see-saw and begin to play. Up and down, up and down. When the pH and pCO_2 are in opposite directions from "normal," the status is respiratory (respiratory = opposite).

Phonetia tires of playing with Paco and runs off to join Carbo who is on a swing. Both go up and both go down, always together. When pH and HCO_3 are either both up or both down, the status is metabolic (metabolic = equal).

$$pH > 7.45 = alkalosis$$
$$pH < 7.35 = acidosis$$

(Turn page for compensatory mechanisms)

Reprinted with permission from Creative Educators, Jefferson, LA

ACID-BASE

R espiratory

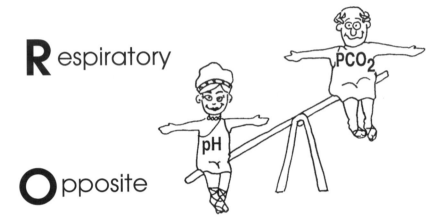

O pposite

M etabolic

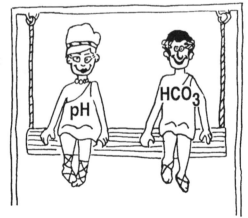

E qual

Reprinted with permission
©1994 Creative Educators

COMPENSATORY MECHANISMS

(This will make more sense to you if you first refer to ACID-BASE STATUS.)

Compensation occurs in respiratory situations when Carbo gets mad at Phonetia for playing with Paco and hops on Paco's side of the see-saw! Imagine all three on the same see-saw.

Compensation occurs in metabolic situations when Paco decides to crash the swinging twosome and hops on with Phonetia and Carbo. Now all go up or all go down.

Reprinted with permission from Creative Educators.

COMPENSATORY MECHANISMS

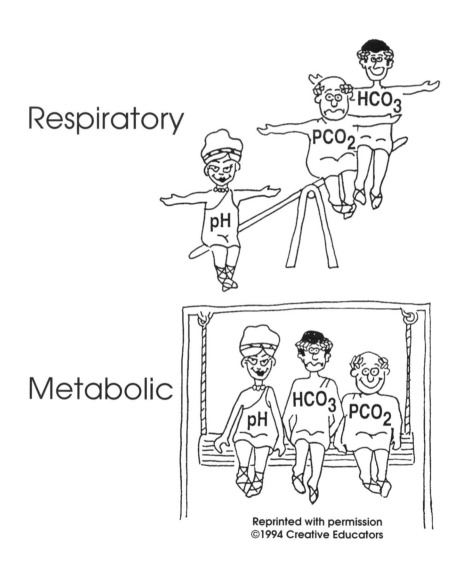

Respiratory

Metabolic

Reprinted with permission
©1994 Creative Educators

ACID-BASE

This referee is calling the shots in Acid-Base. He will help you remember if **ACID** or **BASE** is lost. Think, **A**bove the waist **A**cid is lost. **B**elow the waist **B**ase is lost. The stomach, above the waist, contains HCl (H^+ is an acid). HCl acid is lost during vomiting or when the client has a nasogastric tube. As a result, the client may develop a problem with alkalosis. When a client is hyperventilating, he increases the loss of carbon dioxide which also results in alkalosis.

The bowel below the waist contains alkaline substances which are lost during diarrhea. If alkali are lost, then the client may become acidotic.

There's a BIG exception here! Deep, prolonged vomiting will reach below the waist and lose alkaline intestinal juices resulting in a ketoacidotic state.

CALLING THE SHOTS IN
ACID VS. BASE

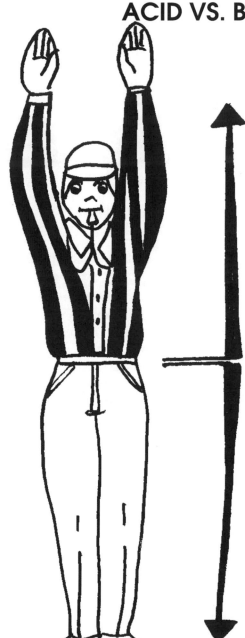

ABOVE

ACID

BELOW

BASE

SHOCK

When you think about the pathophysiology of shock, the classifications (except cardiogenic) have the common bond of decreased venous return (DVR).

HYPOVOLEMIC SHOCK (Hemorrhagic)–If an arm is cut off, that blood is certainly not returning to the heart. DVR! Another example of hypovolemic shock is the guy decides to roof his house on the 4th of July, and sweats out his volume, resulting in dehydration. Less blood to pump = DVR!

NEUROGENIC SHOCK–A severed spinal cord from a gunshot wound or fall allows blood to pool. Nerves have been cut; there is less venous constriction due to absent nerve stimulation.   Spinal anesthesia and barbiturate overdose will cause the same response.

SEPTIC SHOCK (toxic)–An overwhelming infection; generally gram negative organisms will cause a dilation of the blood vessels resulting in a DVR.

VASOGENIC SHOCK (anaphylactic)–A DVR results from an antigen-antibody reaction with release of histamine. Blood that pools causes DVR! Less blood to pump = DVR!

(Refer to **Shock Interventions**.)

In contrast, CARDIOGENIC SHOCK is volume overload NOT volume deficit.

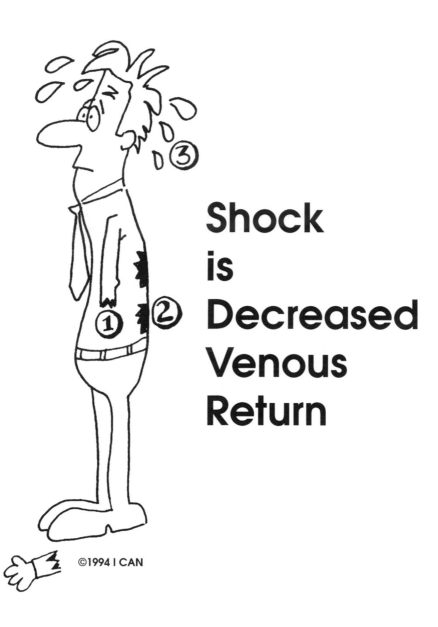

Shock
is
Decreased
Venous
Return

©1994 I CAN

except Cardiogenic

HELP STAMP OUT SHOCK

S *SOLUTIONS* add volume and will increase venous return. Increase the rate. A combination of fluids, blood and plasma expanders (dextran, plasma and albumin) are commonly used. Watch for I.V.s with meds in them. We wouldn't want to turn up the I.V. rate of Pitocin!

H *HEMODYNAMICS* are a way to measure potential shock and evaluate interventions. CVP–(normal is a lucky 7) low CVP means DVR, (decreased venous return) or fluid deficit. Elevated CVP means fluid overload as seen in cardiogenic shock. Low BP reading is one parameter that spells trouble.
*Monitor it every few minutes. As meds are given to increase the BP, it will come up.

O *OXYGEN* will saturate those red blood cells and decrease tissue starvation.

C *CHECK* the skin which is often cold and clammy.

K *KICK* up those feet and legs! There's a lot of blood volume in those legs. Elevate them and let gravity help increase venous return. Don't put the head down. Trendelenburg position may increase cranial pressure, ocular pressure and pressure on the diaphragm.

HELP STAMP OUT SHOCK

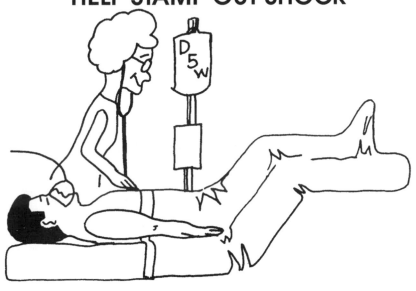

©1994 I CAN

Solutions

Hemodynamics

Oxygen

Checking

Kick 'em up

LUNG SOUNDS

Just breathing in and out makes a normal lung sound that can be heard with a stethoscope. Listen to both sides of the chest because the right side can have clear lung sounds while the left side can have "rales," "wheezes" or some adventitious breath sounds. Listen to the anterior (front) and posterior (back) sounds. How do we know if we hear rales? Rales, sounding like Rice Krispies doing "snap, crackle and pop," are most commonly heard around alveolar sacs more distal to the bronchial tubes. Rales have also been compared to the fizzling of a carbonated drink and are usually heard midway through the inspiratory phase. Wheezes are most often found over the midline or bronchi indicating constriction. Wheezes are continuous sounds, although they are heard more on expiration. Imagine hearing a whistle blow! This is similar to a wheeze.

The bottom line is that breath sounds should be clear and air should be heard moving on both inspiration and expiration. The key is to know what the normal is, so you can detect a difference.

ABNORMAL LUNG SOUNDS

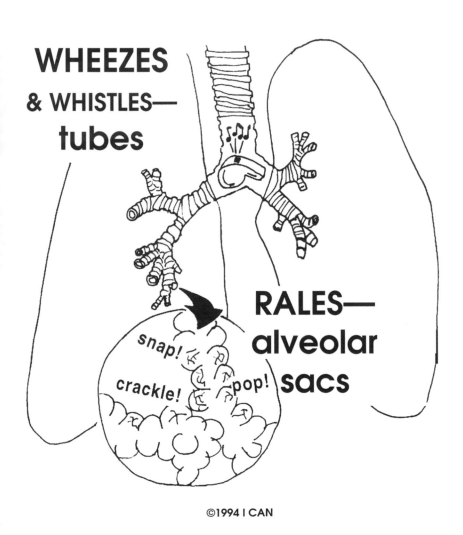

WHEEZES
& WHISTLES—
tubes

RALES—
alveolar
sacs

snap!

crackle!

pop!

©1994 I CAN

"PINK PUFFER": COPD

This guy has COPD, chronic obstructive pulmonary disease. If we could look inside his lungs, we would see a loss of alveolar elasticity, distention and destruction of alveoli. There would be a severe impairment of gas exchange across the alveolar membrane. He is labeled **"PINK PUFFER"** because there is generally no cyanosis. The assessments can be seen in the image on the next page. It is obvious that he has a barrel chest, clubbing of the fingers, thin in appearance, fatigue, pursed-lip breathing, orthopnea and dyspnea. (Refer to **COPD** for nursing care.)

"PINK PUFFER":
Chronic Obstructive
Pulmonary Disease

No cyanosis
Pink (Increased
CO$_2$ retention)

Frequent respiratory
infections

Wheezing

Barrel chest

Fatigues
easily

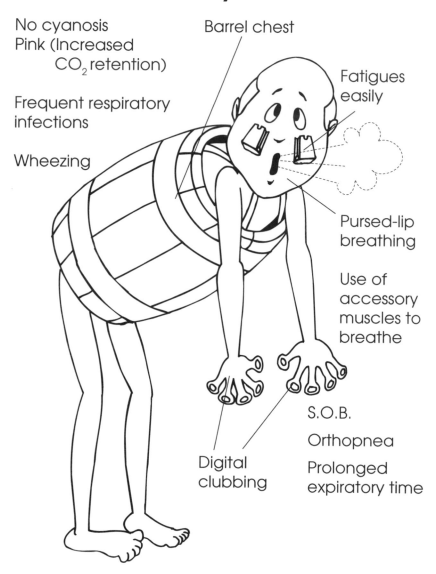

Pursed-lip
breathing

Use of
accessory
muscles to
breathe

S.O.B.

Orthopnea

Prolonged
expiratory time

Digital
clubbing

COPD

Chronic Obstructive Pulmonary Disease is referred to as emphysema. A major risk factor is cigarette smoking.

C   *COUGH* is chronic and nonproductive making it hard to breathe or rest well. A chest x-ray is often ordered to confirm the diagnosis and to look for pneumonia. Nope, one does not have to be NPO for a chest x-ray.

O   *OXYGEN* starvation demands oxygen. A good rule of thumb for the O_2 flow is 2-4 liters. High concentrations of oxygen depress the drive to breathe and cause respiratory distress. ABG's (arterial blood gases) are an excellent way to measure what's happening.

P   *PULMONARY FUNCTION TEST* shows a decrease in lung function possibly calling for postural drainage to reduce secretions and increase oxygen exchange.

D   *DON'T* smoke is probably excellent advice. Emotional support usually helps; nagging doesn't. Drugs and other stuff often given for **COPD** are included on the next page.

CHRONIC OBSTRUCTIVE PULMONARY DISEASE

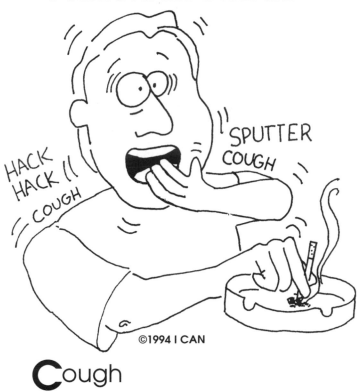

Cough

Oxygen and ABG's

Pulmonary function and postural drainage

Don't smoke

INTERVENTIONS FOR COPD (CHRONIC OBSTRUCTIVE PULMONARY DISEASE)

Since our primary objective for these clients is to enhance oxygen exchange, it makes sense to look at these medicines around the **ABC**'s.

A   *AMINOPHYLLINE* – Relaxes the smooth muscle of the bronchial vessels. (Refer to **Aminophylline Toxicity**.)

B   *BRONCHODILATORS* – Epinephrine (adrenalin) is also used to relax smooth muscle of bronchials. Do not use if client has hypertension or cardiac arrhythmias.

C   *CHEST PHYSIOTHERAPY* – Help remove secretions from the lungs. (Refer to **Postural Drainage.**)

D   *DELIVER OXYGEN AT 2 to 4 LITERS* – High concentrations of oxygen would eliminate the client's hypoxic drive and cause respiratory distress.

E   *EXPECTORANTS* – These will assist in decreasing the viscosity of the mucous.

F   *FORCE FLUIDS* – Fluids will facilitate the removal of secretions.

INTERVENTIONS FOR COPD
(A B C's)

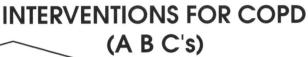

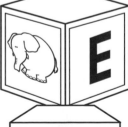**A** minophylline

B ronchodilators

C hest physiotherapy

D eliver oxygen at 2 to 4 liters

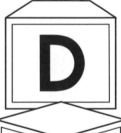**E** xpectorants

F orce fluids

AMINOPHYLLINE TOXICITY

Aminophylline (bronchodilator) is a wonderful and effective drug that relaxes and expands the bronchi reversing airway obstruction. This drug is commonly used in clients with problems such as: asthma, croup, chronic bronchitis and COPD.

Meet **AMILY TOXICITY** who received too much of this drug. We recommend that you stay out of her way! When she gets too much of this wonder drug, she **THROWS UP**! (Notice she has her hands covering her mouth.) Amily has an "A" on her shirt for "**hyperACTIVITY**". When the level gets high, Amily starts bouncing off the walls. The "**T**" on her shirt is for "**TACHYCARDIA**". Amily is so active that her heart rate must race (tachycardia) to keep up with her.

The therapeutic range for aminophylline levels is 10-20 mcg/ml.

*Keep your eyes open, and your assessments will tell you the story about the effectiveness of this drug. If signs of toxicity occur, report to the physician and check the TBL.

AMINOPHYLLINE TOXICITY

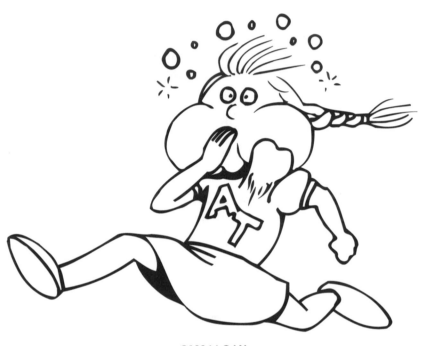

©1994 I CAN

Amily Toxicity

CYSTIC FIBROSIS

This little guy is a "Sicker Kid". His disease is inherited from an autosomal recessive trait. The exocrine glands that normally produce the enzymes lipase (digests fats), trypsin (digests protein) and amylase (digests starches) are not functioning normally. He's doing without a good part of his nutrition (about 40% of his food gets ingested). The other issue is that cystic fibrosis causes these enzymes to become so tenacious that they cause other problems. Organs affected by this disease include the lungs, pancreas, GI tract, and liver. **"Sicker Kid"** will assist you in remembering the major concepts in cystic fibrosis.

S   *STEATORRHEA* (fat in stool) smelly stools with increased amount. **SWEAT TEST** indicating high salt content may be diagnostic. Adequate salt intake is important.

I   *ILEUS-MECONIUM* may be present in newborns. The small intestine is blocked with thick mucous causing symptoms of intestinal obstruction.

C   *CONSTANT* **hunger** because of poor food absorption.

K   *VITAMINS K,A,D,E* (fat soluble) may be supplemented.

E   *ENZYME* **(pancreatic) replacement** is mandatory. Administer prior to meals and snacks.

R   *REDUCE* dietary fat. Use **low fat** milk.

K   *KEEP* **calories up.** Use **simple sugars** as a source of energy.

I   *INFECTION* may be a way of life, especially respiratory infections due to pulmonary congestion. Administer oxygen and IV fluids to keep secretions thin.

D   *DRINK* **plenty of fluids** to prevent dehydration and to keep mucous thin. DIET high in calorie, high protein, fats as tolerated or decreased, and increase salt intake.

CYSTIC FIBROSIS

S teatorrhea
S weat test

I leus-meconium

C onstant hunger

K vitamins

E nzyme replacement

R educe fat

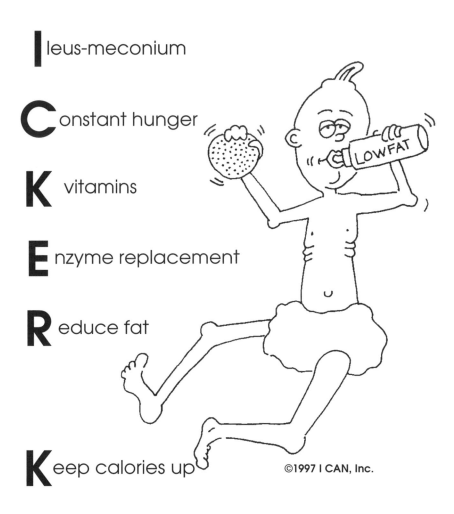

©1997 I CAN, Inc.

K eep calories up

I nfection

D rink plenty of fluids

"BLUE BLOATER": CHRONIC BRONCHITIS

Meet Ol' Blue the dog, who has bronchitis. He has an increase in mucus production with a major amount of inflammation and narrowing of the airway passages. When you listen to his breath sounds, expect to hear *expiratory wheezing*.

Due to his *cyanosis* and polycythemia which gives the skin a characteristic color, Ol' Blue may be labeled as "**BLUE BLOATER**." Notice his position in bed; high-Fowler's which will optimize the expansion of his lungs. The IV will also deliver the necessary bronchodilator (aminophylline) to assist in the breathing and *shortness of breath*. Monitor the theophylline level (TBL) for toxicity. Ol' Blue will get *restless* if he is experiencing *S.O.B.* or if his TBL gets too high. (Refer to **Aminophylline Toxicity** for more specific information.)

If we were to look under the covers, we would observe him using his accessory muscles to breathe. His vital signs reveal an elevated respiratory rate and prolonged expiratory time. Get him those Kleenex for all of that sputum he is coughing. It should not be discolored unless he has an infection. Let the poor dog REST!

"BLUE BLOATER":
Chronic Bronchitis

Productive cough
Hypoxia
Expiratory wheezing
Cyanotic nail beds
Restless
S. O. B.
Tachypnea
Acidosis
Hypercapnia

AMINOPHYLLINE

PULMONARY EDEMA

This condition is a result of too much fluid in the lung, both in the interstitial and in the alveolar spaces. Pulmonary edema results from severe impairment of the left heart function. **MAD DOG** COMES TO THE RESCUE!

M *MORPHINE* will decrease preload, allowing blood to pool in the extremities. As a result, the heart will not work as hard. A major problem is anxiety, due to feeling they are drowning in their secretions. Although morphine will decrease the anxiety, monitor for potential respiratory depression.

A *AMINOPHYLLINE* will decrease shortness of breath by expanding the bronchi. (Refer to **Aminophylline Toxicity** for more specific information.)

D *DIGOXIN* slows heart rate by increasing cardiac output. Hold med if apical heart rate below 60. Therapeutic level is 0.6-2.0 mg/ml; above 2.0 mg/ml is toxic. Signs of toxicity are anorexia, nausea, vomiting, headache, fatigue, bradycardia and photophobia.

D *DIURETICS*, especially Lasix dump the fluid overload through the kidneys. Monitor potassium level. Hypokalemia precipitates digitalis toxicity. (Therapeutic level of potassium is 3.5-5.0 mEq/L.) Daily weight will help evaluate the fluid loss along with an accurate intake and output record.

O *OXYGEN* is given to saturate red blood cells and provide more oxygen to the tissues. Oxygen is usually given via nasal cannula.

G *GASES* are evaluated to maintain pH, PO_2 and PCO_2 within appropriate limits. (Refer to **Acid-Base**.)

PULMONARY EDEMA

Morphine

Aminophylline

Digoxin

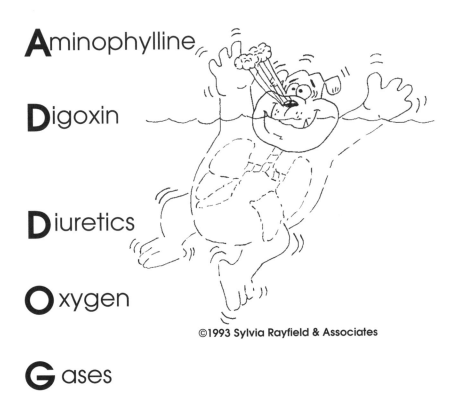

Diuretics

Oxygen

©1993 Sylvia Rayfield & Associates

Gases

POSTURAL DRAINAGE

To remove secretions from the upper lung fields (RUL and LUL), place the client in the upright position. To get secretions to drain out of the lower lobes, stand them on their heads (not literally). Trendelenburg's position will facilitate the removal of secretions. To affect the RML, position client on the left side with the head slanted down. To remove the secretions from the lingula LL, place client on the right side with the head slanted down.

Postural drainage will be done with clients who have COPD (chronic obstructive pulmonary disease), pneumonia and bronchitis. (Just to name a few!)

POSTURAL DRAINAGE

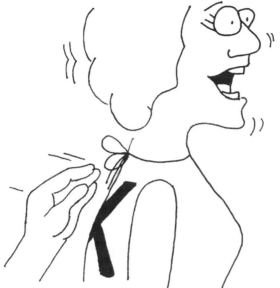

draining upper lung

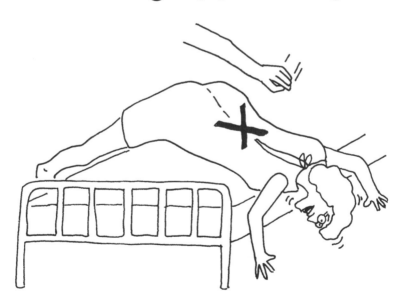

draining lower lung

VENTILATOR CARE

This poor guy has found himself on a ventilator. To accurately evaluate the effectiveness of the vent, closely VIEW the client's ARTERIAL BLOOD GASES. Pressure should be maintained at the puncture site for a minimum of 5 minutes. After changing any ventilatory settings or suctioning the client, wait for 30 minutes to draw the ABG's. After procedures, carefully evaluate client's vital signs, pulse oximetry, color, etc., and check that VENT alarms are on. To determine the adequacy of air exchange, EVALUATE the BREATH SOUNDS. Look for equal chest movement, client's color and respirations. Calmly explain equipment and alarms to both the client and family. Ventilators are such a scary proposition that people become stressed. NOTICE GI COMPLICATIONS from potential STRESS ULCERS. The majority of clients will require cimetidine (tagamet).

Once clients are dependent on a ventilator, it is not easy to get them off. Usually, TWENTY PERCENT have to stay on until the plug is pulled. The other 80% do quite well especially if they are weaned slowly. Weaning is done best during the day time hours. Hold morphine or valium while weaning.

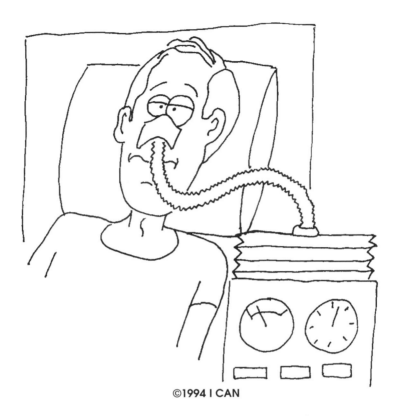

©1994 I CAN

View ABG's

Evaluate breath sounds

Notice G.I. complications (stress ulcer)

Twenty % can't be weaned; wean slowly

TUBERCULOSIS SKIN TEST

Multi- drug resistant tuberculosis is persistent and may present a severe threat to the general public health. People with suppressed immune systems, such as those with AIDS and the elderly are at a particular risk. A tuberculin skin test is used for screening. A small amount (0.1 ml) of purified protein derivative (PPD) is injected into the intradermal tissue using a tuberculin syringe equipped with a small gauge (such as a 25 ga.) needle. The intradermal (intracutaneous) injection is made by injecting the end of the needle just below the surface of the skin. The needle bevel side should be up. This process will assist in raising a "wheal."

Look at the injection site of the "wheal" in 48 and 72 hours. If the wheal is red and raised by 10 mm, the reading is considered positive. A positive reaction means the individual has at some time been exposed to the TB bacilli and has developed antibodies. It does not mean that the person has an active TB infection. Further evaluation with a chest x-ray may demonstrate the presence of calcified lesions. If active TB is suspected, bacteriologic studies may be done to identify acid-fast bacilli.

TB
✓ at
48 and 72 hours

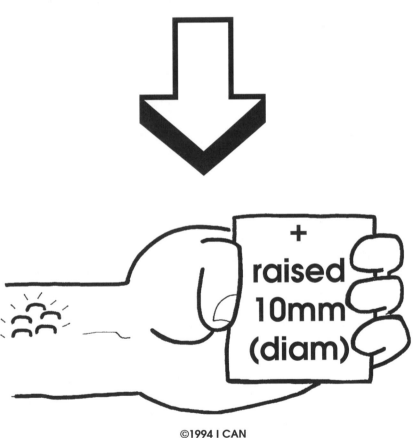

TUBERCULOSIS

INA has the typical signs and symptoms of tuberculosis including fatigue, weight loss, anorexia, chronic productive cough, night sweats, and hemoptysis (advanced stage). In order to help the *mycobacterium tuberculosis* **rise** out of her, there are several medications which may be prescribed. **"RISE"** will assist in remembering these medications.

R   *RIFAMPIN* - This medication is most often prescribed with isoniazid (INH). The secretions (sweat, urine) may turn orange. Hepatitis may be a complication, especially in alcoholics. Rifampin should be administered once daily on an empty stomach.

I   *ISONIAZID* **(INH)** - This is the primary medication used in prophylactic treatment of tuberculosis. Adverse reactions include hepatitis, and / or hepatotoxicity. Peripheral neuropathies can be prevented by pretreating with pyridoxine (vitamin B6). INH should be administered once daily on an empty stomach.

S   *STREPTOMYCIN* - Two major adverse effects from this medication are ototoxicity and nephrotoxicity. Due to the susceptibility to cranial nerve VIII, this medication is generally avoided in the elderly. Use it with caution if clients have renal disease. Hearing must be evaluated frequently. Streptomycin may not be given po.

E   *EHAMBUTOL* - This medication is frequently administered with rifampin and INH. Assess vision prior to therapy to identify side effects of optic neuritis which may result in loss of central vision from this medication. Ethambutol should be administered once daily with food or meals to decrease gastric irritation.

INA TUBERCULOSIS

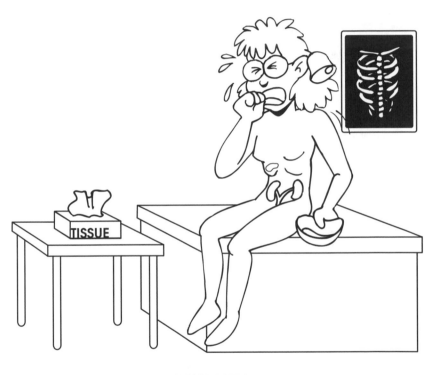

AMPHOTERICIN B (FUNGIZONE)

Amphotericin B commonly given IV in a distal vein (watch for thrombosis) is a very potent and toxic drug. It may also be given orally. It is given to clients with histoplasmosis (a fungus infection of the lung) to disrupt the plasma membrane and destroy the fungal cells. It should be mixed only with water and not saline and should be slowly infused as rapid infusion may cause cardiovascular collapse. It should not be mixed with other drugs.

The undesirable effect of **nephrotoxicity** can be reduced by hydrating the client. Notice the client is on a scale as the **weight** and **intake and output** should be monitored. His BUN **(Blood urea nitrogen), liver enzymes, urinalysis, and electrolytes** should be checked before and during treatment. If the BUN rises, the drug may have to be discontinued to prevent further destruction of the liver.

AMPHOTERICIN B
(FUNGIZONE)

A mphotericin

N

T

I

F

U

N

G

A

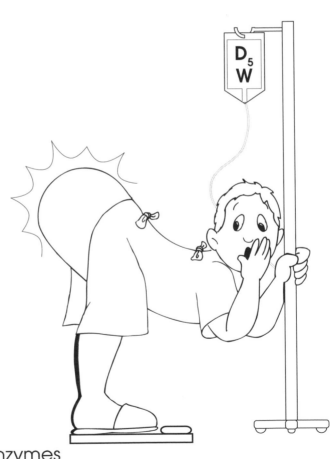

L iver enzymes
ytes

FLUID VOLUME STATUS

The arrow indicates that fluid (plasma) volume decreases during dehydration. This will cause an increase in the sodium blood level above the normal range of 135-145 meq/L. The hematocrit will also rise (above 45%) due to the same principle.

The opposite occurs during pregnancy. Due to increased fluid (plasma) levels, the hematocrit and the serum sodium levels decrease. This dilution of the red blood cells is referred to as pseudoanemia. Evaluation of the serum sodium and hematocrit levels are excellent indicators of the fluid volume status. Several important nursing interventions for these clients include: daily weights, intake and output records, specific gravity evaluation of the urine, assessing the skin turgor, and lips and mucous membranes. An important assessment for infants regarding their fluid status is to observe if the fontanels are depressed or bulging.

This is an excellent tool to assist you in remembering the concept of the fluid volume status.

FLUID VOLUME STATUS

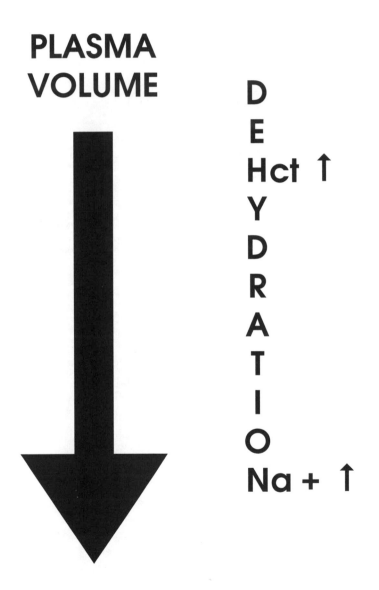

PLASMA VOLUME

DEHYDRATION

Hct ↑

Na + ↑

FLUID SHIFTS

Fluid shifts are easier to figure out if you remember this nursery rhyme:

> "Mary had a little lamb and everywhere Mary went, the lamb was sure to go." Mary is salt (NaCl), and the lamb is water. Everywhere salt goes, water follows.

You may be asking yourself, how does this fit in with my nursing care? Frequently, we need to do health teaching for clients who are taking certain medications. The group that comes to our mind are the thiazides. Would we want these individuals eating a high sodium diet? Of course not! That would defeat the purpose for these diuretics.

Diuretics are given to remove fluid from the body. If we increase the sodium intake for these clients, they will continue to retain fluid. Everywhere salt (NaCl) goes, water follows.

FLUID SHIFTS

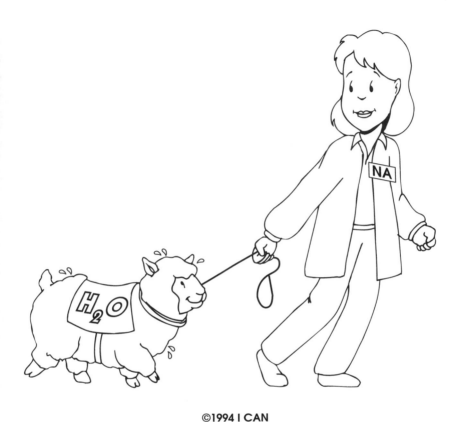

©1994 I CAN

"Mary had a little lamb and everywhere Mary went the lamb was sure to go."

RENAL

This system can be quite simple when you compare it to a water faucet and pitcher as we have on the image page. In the normal (healthy) faucet, the flow is great. There is no obstruction, and the filter is fine.

Notice in the **PRERENAL** diagram, there is decrease in the flow of water (urine). There is faucet (renal) ischemia–a decrease in the water pressure. Have you ever tried getting hot water out of the faucet while the dish washer is on? This can occur in the renal system from hemorrhage, shock, burns or decreased cardiac output.

In the **INTRARENAL** diagram, there is decreased output and some WBC's and protein which do not normally belong in the urine. This is due to kidney tissue pathology. In the faucet, it is as if someone came along and cut an opening in the filter on the spicket. This may be from glomerulonephritis, pyelonephritis, severe crushing injury, chemicals or medications.

In the **POSTRENAL** diagram, there is an obstruction in the water flow. This could be from the lime build up in the system which is causing a decrease in the free fluid. This is exactly what happens in the renal system. Some examples are: urinary calculi, benign prostatic hypertrophy (BPH) and cancer.

Remember to check renal function tests, BUN 10–20, creatinine .5–1.5. As the renal function decreases, these values will increase.

RENAL

Normal

50–60cc

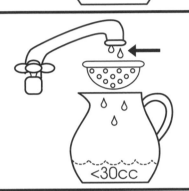

Prerenal

<30cc

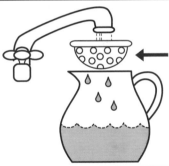

Intrarenal

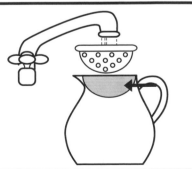

Postrenal

AMINOGLYCOSIDES

These images illustrate two of the major side effects of these drugs.

Ototoxicity–Hearing loss may be irreversible.

Nephrotoxicity–Oliguria may lead to kidney damage.

AMINOGLYCOSIDES

Gentamycin
Kanamycin Sulfate
Neomycin Sulfate
Streptomycin Sulfate

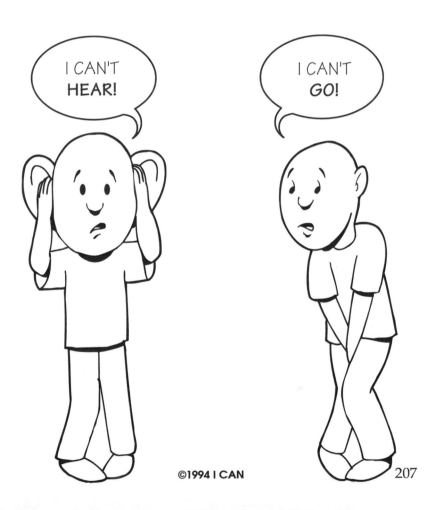

BURNS

Berny has been in a fire, and as you can see, he is wrapped up like a mummy. Berny **BURNS** will help us learn burn care.

B *BREATHING*–Keep airway open. Facial burns, singed nasal hair, hoarseness, sooty sputum, bloody sputum, and labored respirations indicate TROUBLE!
BODY IMAGE–Assist Berny in coping by encouraging expression of thoughts and feelings.

U *URINE OUTPUT* –In an adult, urine output should be 30 to 70 cc per hour, in the child 20 to 50 cc per hour, and in the infant 10 to 20 cc per hour. Watch the K^+ to keep it between 3.5-5.0 mEq/L. Keep the CVP around 12 cm water pressure.

R *RESUSCITATION OF FLUID*–Salt and electrolyte solutions are essential over the first 24 hours. Maintain BP at 90 to 100 systolic. One-half of the fluid for the first 24 hours should be administered over the first 8-hour period, then the remainder is administered over the next 16 hours. First 24-hour calculation starts at the time of injury.
RULE OF NINE –Used for adults to determine burn surface area.

N *NUTRITION*–Protein and calories are components of the diet. Supplemental gastric tube feedings or hyperalimentation may be used in clients with large burned areas. Daily weights will assist in evaluating the nutritional needs.

S *SHOCK*–Watch the BP, CVP and renal function.
SILVADENE–For infection.

REMEMBER THESE PEOPLE ARE AFRAID AND NEED SUPPORT!

BURNS

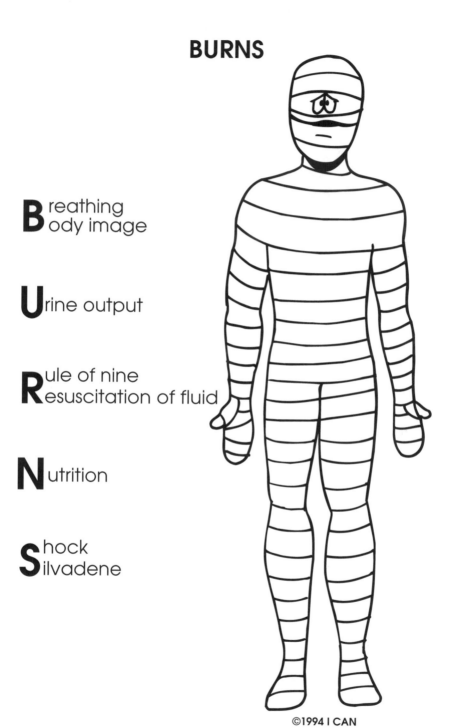

B reathing
B ody image

U rine output

R ule of nine
R esuscitation of fluid

N utrition

S hock
S ilvadene

©1994 I CAN

CARE OF CLIENT AFTER MASTECTOMY

Have you ever had a chicken without a breast? Well, this may be a first for you. Meet "Ester the breastless chicken." Ester had a mastectomy due to cancer. She has a family history with both her mother and sister having breast cancer. She refused to have the recommended mammogram every 1 to 2 years after she turned 40.

After her mastectomy, no *BLOOD PRESSURES* or lab sticks were done on the affected side. She maintained the affected side in an *ELEVATED* position. Each joint was to be elevated and positioned higher than the more proximal joint to promote drainage. Ester met some wonderful women from *REACH FOR RECOVERY* who provided her with support. She was given pamphlets to read and phone numbers of some contact people who also had a mastectomy. After they left, she started her *EXTENSION* and *FLEXION* exercises. Squeezing a ball is a great exercise. **ABDUCTION** and **EXTERNAL** rotation should not be the initial exercises. Ester was taught how to do a **SBE** (self breast examination) once a month. The nurse recommended that she do it while she was taking her shower. The staff encouraged Ester to discuss her fears, concerns and anxieties in order **TO PROMOTE A POSITIVE SELF IMAGE**.

CARE OF CLIENT AFTER MASTECTOMY

BP—not on affected side

Reach for Recovery

Elevate affected side
xtension and flexion
    exercises—initially
    (squeeze a ball)

A bduction and external
    rotation should not
    be initial exercise

S B E—once a month—
    about one week after
    period

©1994 I CAN

To promote a positive self image

MENOPAUSE

MINNIE wakes up nights, throwing off those covers and finding herself wet with sweat from a hot flash. She reaches for her estrogen (premarin) with one hand since it will help control these night sweats and her heart shaped fan with the other. Her fan will cool her down, and it is heart shaped because during this time in her life she may wear her heart on her sleeve. She can be very sensitive and moody during menopause and small comments hurt her feelings. The estrogen will also improve Minnie's lipid profile and will decrease risks to her heart. (Refer to Josephine Bone-A-Part for more detail regarding estrogen.)

Vaginal BLEEDING seems to increase at menstrual period times and MINNIE must always be prepared with "supplies" because she can never tell when that period will show up. Excessive bleeding leads to ANEMIA and now she's got to take iron along with her other drugs, herbs and teas that reduce these "NO FUN symptoms".

Remember–This "PAUSE" is not a brief time in one's life and cannot be fixed quickly. Often symptoms persist for 3+ years!

MINNIE PAUSE

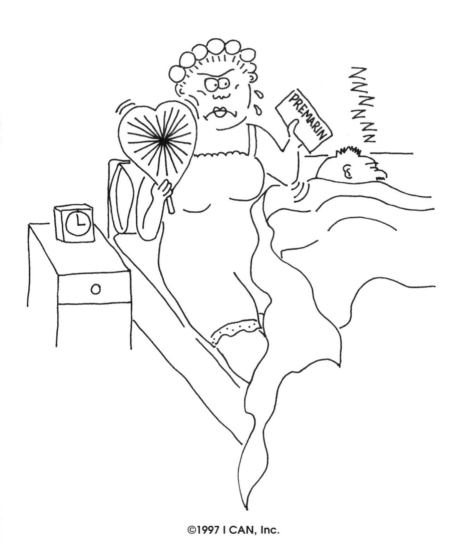

BENIGN PROSTATE HYPERTROPHY

The poor guy who has his "tubes" squeezed tightly due to an enlarged prostate gland will likely find himself going to surgery for a transurethral resection of the prostate (TURP). Prostatic tissue is removed through a resectoscope, so the urethra can once again pass urine easily.

When the guy comes back from surgery, he will likely have a triple lumen tube in his bladder to maintain continuous bladder irrigation (CBI) or Murphy drip. The *TUBE* will provide for *URINARY OUTPUT*, but it will contain bright *RED DRAINAGE*. If you see pieces of clots in the tube, it's time to increase the CBI to wash out the clots. Retained blood *CLOTS* may cause hemorrhage and we do not want that to happen! Unfortunately CLOTS may also cause bladder *SPASMS* that hurt. Belladonna and opium suppositories (B&O) are often ordered to help relieve the spasms. If the client complains of pain, evaluate the urinary drainage and make sure the catheter is patent.

Obstructions most commonly occur in the initial 24 hours due to clots in the bladder. Overdistention of the bladder can precipitate hemorrhage as well as bladder spasms.

TURPS

Tubes

Urinary output

Red drainage

Pieces of clots

Spasms

©1994 I CAN

SAFETY WITH RADIUM IMPLANTS

"How do you feel today" is adopted from Sue Crow's book *Asepsis, The Right Touch*, an excellent down to earth book on infection control. Let's assume that the character in the bed has a radium implant.

We want to plan our nursing care from afar! When you are in very close proximity to the client who has a radium implant, you get almost as much radiation as they do. Talk to them from as much DISTANCE as you can manage. Except when giving direct care, attempt to maintain distance of six feet from the source of radiation. Plan your care, so that you are in close proximity for the shortest period of TIME.

Some institutions provide lead SHIELDING; generally not necessary if time and distance principles are observed.

Remember, these clients will get lonely because they are on bedrest and can't leave their room. *Be sure they can reach the telephone and the call light!*

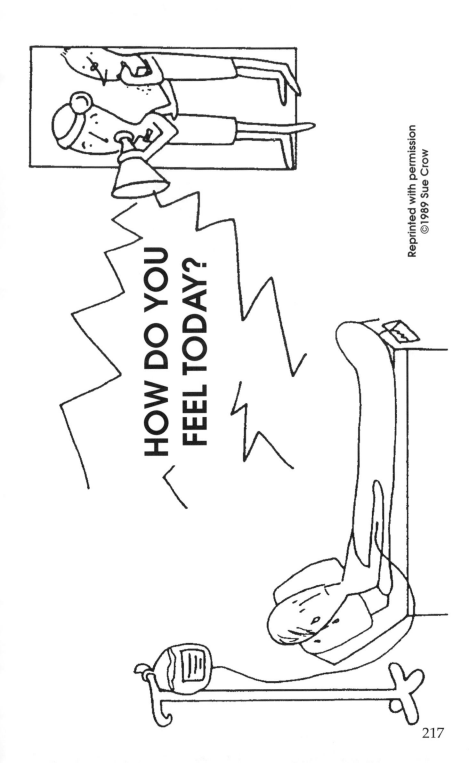

217

EXTERNAL RADIATION

Sammy Shade is receiving external radiation for cancer. This source of radiation is directed toward the area of the tumor and draining lymphatics. He is likely to experience *SEVERE NAUSEA AND VOMITING, HEMATURIA* and *DIARRHEA*. Meticulous oral hygiene is important to decrease complications associated with vomiting. Antidiarrheal medications, low residue, high protein and a bland diet will decrease complications of diarrhea. Notice, Sammy has no hair on his head, very little on his face and probably none in his pubic area. Sammy will need help to cope with changes in his body image due to **ALOPECIA**. He may decide to wear a wig or turban. Sammy needs to pat, not rub, hair dry after shampooing to avoid excessive handling of brittle hair. Ice packs to the scalp may reduce hair loss. *ANEMIA* is a common side effect of therapy. Maintain adequate rest in between scheduled activities. Evaluate Sammy for signs of hypoxia. Encourage a diet high in protein, vitamins and iron. Assess for signs of infection and bleeding. External radiation is prone to **DRY THE SKIN** particularly *EVALUATE* the site of radiation. This site may remain photophobic, so let's advise Sammy to remain in the **SHADE**.

EXTERNAL RADIATION

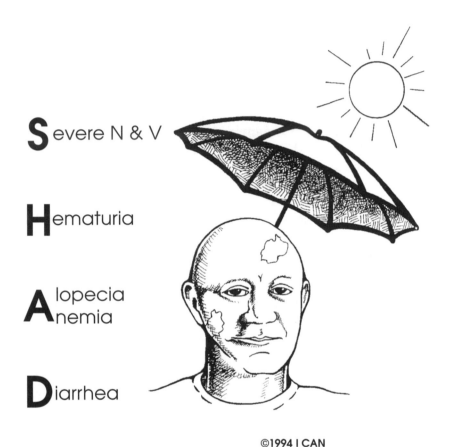

Severe N & V

Hematuria

Alopecia
Anemia

Diarrhea

©1994 I CAN

Evaluate skin for redness/dryness

TREATMENT OF ULCERATIVE COLITIS AND CROHN'S

Cathy Crampy has inflammatory bowel disease. She is bent over with the **CRAMPS** due to the inflammation. This is treated with steroids and a low fat and low fiber diet. Poor Cathy has her legs together to hold in that *DIARRHEA*. She is taking some antidiarrheal medications to decrease this problem.

Her *PAIN* is being relieved through her diet, *ANTICHOLINERGICS* and corticosteroids. Cathy may be NPO to decrease bowel activity; *FLUIDS* are introduced gradually. She will receive IV fluids and may even require hyperalimentation to restore the deficiencies.

Sulfasalazine (AZULFIDINE) is one of the *ANTIMICROBIALS* used to prevent exacerbations.

Her *MEALS* are modified to correct the deficiencies. She is on a high protein, high caloric and high vitamin diet. Cathy may live a very stressful life. She is always a day behind her deadlines.

COUNSELING will help her to identify how this life style can contribute to this condition. Emotional *SUPPORT* will assist Cathy Crampy in decreasing the stress in her life and help her to learn "To slow down and stop and smell the flowers in life."

TREATMENT OF ULCERATIVE COLITIS AND CROHN'S

Control diarrhea
Control inflammation

Relieve pain
Restore fluid

Anticholinergics
Antimicrobials

Meals—correct
nutritional deficiencies

Psychological counseling

Support emotionally/coping

©1994 I CAN

COLOSTOMY

Clients with ulcerative colitis, Crohn's disease or other disease process in the lower gastrointestinal tract may require surgery that brings fecal elimination to an opening on the outside of the abdominal wall.

Connie Colostomy says that her colostomy is just like her ANUS.

A *ABLE* to regulate her stool through regular irrigations; therefore a colostomy bag is not required. Irrigations should be the same time frame daily.

N *NOT* watery. The stools are formed and do not leak on her clothes.

U *U* can do all you can do without the colostomy. Some foods will liquefy stools or cause noisy problems.

S *SWIMMING* is OK! Showers and tub baths are also acceptable.

This is probably NOT the case for Connie's friend ILLE who has an ileostomy.

Ille's stool is liquid. Bags are attached to the skin and skin breaks down easily. She must be taught about cleaning, removing the adhesive that holds the bag in place and cleanliness of the bag. She is usually not able to regulate the ileostomy because it is watery. She may lose fluids and electrolytes and need replacement. Some foods may also cause noisy (flatus) and "smelly" problems for Ille, which is embarrassing and hard to control.

Remember—Both Connie and Ille will have to live with these ostomys. The nurse's best approach is psychological support and education. They will need support through excellent therapeutic communication. The more they know about caring for themselves, the more "normal" they can be.

CONNIE COLOSTOMY

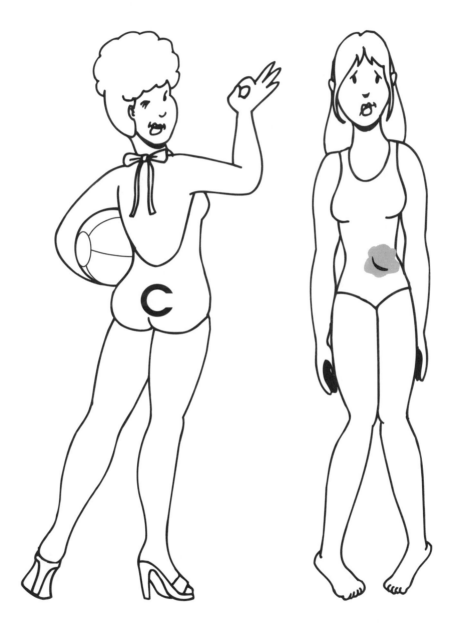

CONNIE COLOSTOMY   **ILLE OSTOMY**

PEPTIC ULCER DISEASE

Old **PUD** is a fine specimen of a man. He's standing there tapping his foot waiting impatiently on that bus, smoking his cigarette with a vengeance and checking to see if it's time for another NSAID (Nonsteroidal Anti-inflammatory drugs may cause GI bleeding). Just the kind of behavior that might precipitate peptic ulcer disease. When you think ulcers (except stress ulcers), think pain. Imagine a drop of hydrochloric acid on your open hand! First, the hand will hurt or burn, and once the acid has eaten the skin away, the hand will bleed. If the hand could be protected by a glove (food or drugs) the HCL might not eat through enough to bleed.

Drug timing is important in preventing this pain and bleeding. Generally, use anticholinergics before meals. (Refer to **Anticholinergics.**) Tagamet and zantac may be given with or after meals. Consider coating the stomach lining with the "white chalky stuff" such as maalox, titrilac, gelusil, or amphojel 1 hour after meals. Avoid giving within 1 to 2 hours of other medicines. Remind clients on sodium restriction to check the labels for sodium content. Amphojel, titralac, and digel have high sodium content. These clients will also need assistance in dietary modifications.

The Heliocobactor Pylori (Helicopter) organism may be responsible for PUD. Treatment to eradicate the H. pylori may include tetracycline, metronidazole and bismuth subsalicylate (Pepto-Bismol).

ULCERS

Pain

Ulcers bleed

Drug timing

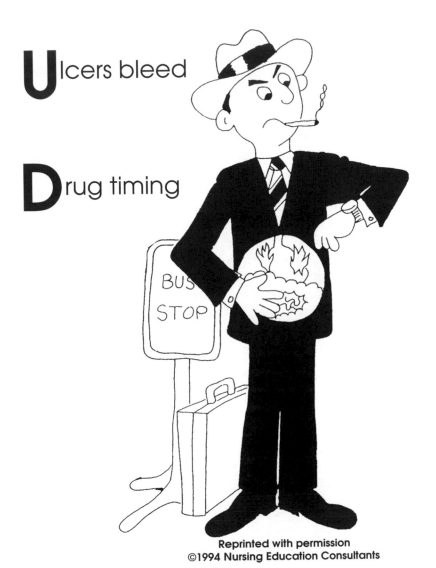

ANTACIDS

Mag has had a history of an ulcer, but feels much better now since antacids coat her stomach lining. She, however, has developed another serious problem with DIARRHEA!!!! This is a major side effect of antacids containing magnesium such as Milk of Magnesia. The diarrhea must get under control or she will need to meet Alkali, a cousin, which will assist her in correcting the metabolic acidosis which may occur as a complication from the diarrhea. **Mag** should be monitored for dehydration, hypokalemia, and hyponatremia. If **Mag** were to remain on magnesium oxide for prolonged therapy, the magnesium level should be monitored periodically.

AL is also in the family and is taking an aluminum antacid such as amphogel for his ulcer symptoms. As you can see, **Al's** problem is constipation. He is so full of it that he can't get rid of it. CONSTIPATION is a major side effect of antacids containing aluminum.

Remember–Teach clients to take antacids one hour after meals and to refrain from taking other oral medications within 1-2 hours of any antacid.

AUNT ACID'S FAMILY

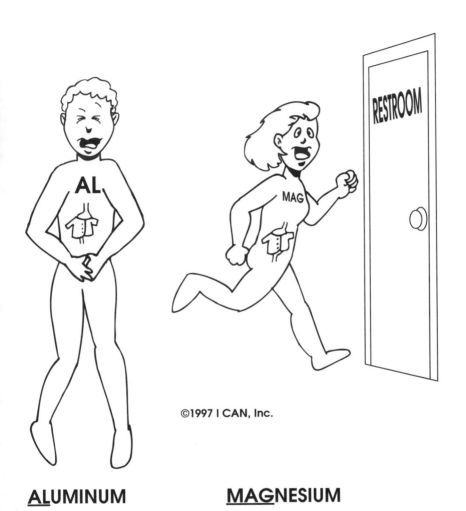

©1997 I CAN, Inc.

ALUMINUM   MAGNESIUM

POSTOPERATIVE GI ASSESSMENT

Back in the operating room as a client is being prepared for abdominal surgery, drapes are used over the body to help maintain sterility. Let's use the word **DRAPES** to look at the concept of postoperative GI assessment.

D *DRESSING*–Evaluate amount and characteristics of drainage.

R *RESPIRATORY SYSTEM*–Listen for those breath sounds! Get in some T, C & DB (turning, coughing and deep breathing) to prevent atelectasis.

A *ABDOMINAL ASSESSMENT*–Watch for abdominal distention. Normal bowel sounds should be heard every 5 to 20 seconds. The abdomen should remain soft. If it becomes hard, this may indicate bleeding, paralytic ileus, or peritonitis. If in doubt, measure abdominal girth.

AMBULATE–Will decrease blood clots caused by pooling of blood in extremities. Will decrease the development of a paralytic ileus.

P *PAIN MEDICINE*–Keep them comfortable. If they have a patient-controlled analgesia (PCA) pump in place, teach them how to use it.
PATENCY OF TUBES–This can be done through irrigations and monitoring the suction of drains and tubes.

E *ELIMINATION*– Keep an I & O record.

S *SPLINT*– Splint abdominal incision during T, C, and DB.

GI ASSESSMENT

Dressing

Respiratory system

Abdominal assessment
Ambulate

Pain medicine
Patency of the tubes

Elimination

Splint

©1994 I CAN

DUMPING SYNDROME

This is a complication that can occur after gastric resection when stomach contents enter the intestine. The image that will pull this concept together for you is the DUMP TRUCK. Imagine that you are in a dump truck on the edge of a mountain. How would you feel? We know we would be nervous as kittens, sweaty and our heart would beat very rapidly. On a mountain edge, we are sure we would be dizzy and very weak. We may also have some abdominal cramping with some distention. These signs are, of course, because we are in the **HIGH** position. (Think of TOO MUCH, TOO SOON = TOO HIGH) Too much carbohydrate, salt, liquid, refined sugar, and in the high position on top of all of that is going to make us (excuse the expression) poop! The gastric contents high in carbohydrates rapidly enter the jejunum.

To remember how to prevent this from occurring, think of the dump truck in the **LOW** position. Think **LOW**. Teach clients to think small (LOW) meals. The carbohydrates, salt intake, and sugar need to be **LOW** (small amounts). No fluids with meals or for one hour following the meal. Lie client down for 20 to 30 minutes after meals to delay stomach emptying.

DUMPING SYNDROME

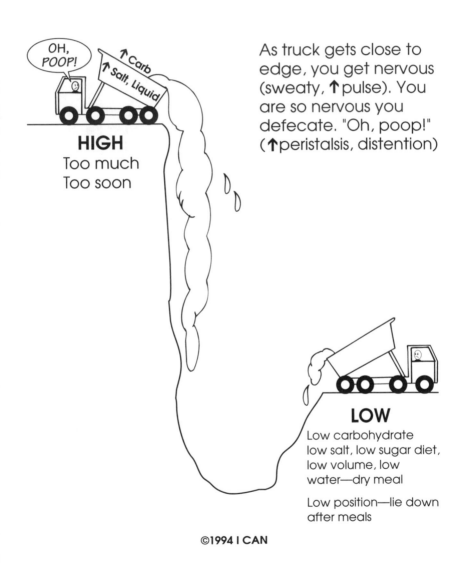

As truck gets close to edge, you get nervous (sweaty, ↑pulse). You are so nervous you defecate. "Oh, poop!" (↑peristalsis, distention)

©1994 I CAN

NASOGASTRIC TUBES

First, think about tubes in general. Remember, fluid or air can flow either way in a tube. In this case, we're looking at the nasogastric tube as a feeding tube to accommodate the passing of fluid. The major safety issue with the N/G tube is PLACE-MENT. We want to know where the end of that tube is prior to putting fluid in. Nothing like dumping a feeding solution into the lung because the tube has become displaced out of the stomach! The feeding solution should be ROOM TEMPERA-TURE before putting into the body. If the client is turned to the RIGHT SIDE during the feeding, the stomach can empty better. USE GRAVITY to allow the solution to run in. Some folks use those big bulb syringes. If that's the case, squeezing the fluid in with the bulb can place undue pressure on the stomach. ASPI-RATE stomach contents prior to administering a feeding. Be sure to return the gastric contents aspirated, otherwise necessary electrolytes will be wasted. Most procedures agree to hold the tube feeding and notify the physician if 100 cc or more are aspirated. *ENDING* the feeding with a little WATER (approxi-mately 30–50 cc) will keep the feeding tube clean. Document this process in the chart.

NG TUBE

Never give without checking

Give warm (room temperature)

Turn to right side

Use gravity

Be sure to aspirate

End with water & chart

ANTICHOLINERGICS

The major side effects of these medications are easily seen on the next page. Some examples of these medications include: Atropine, Methantheline (Banthine), Propantheline (Pro-Banthine), and Dicyclomine hydrochloride (Bentyl). Of course these drugs are given because of the desirable effects of decreasing salivation, lacrimation, urination, diarrhea, and GI motility. Blurred vision and dilated pupils are also side effects. It's when we get too much that we get in trouble.

Remember–These medications are contraindicated in closed and open angle glaucoma, prostatic hypertrophy and obstructive bowel disease.

ANTICHOLINERGIC MEDICATIONS

Can't pee
Can't see
Can't spit
Can't shit

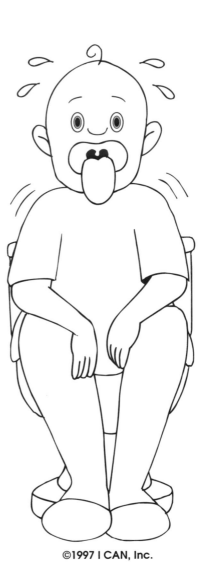

©1997 I CAN, Inc.

CIRRHOSIS

Here is Larry Leak Liver, who is no longer able to synthesize protein. This results in a decreased colloidal osmotic pressure. (COP holds fluid in the liver and blood vessels.) Since he no longer easily accepts blood from his unique dual blood supply, he also develops portal hypertension. This causes poor Larry to Leak fluid into the peritoneal cavity resulting in **ASCITES**. Too much swelling in the esophagus will cause Larry to get into *AIRWAY* trouble. To prevent complications from *SWELLING*, he may be started on diuretics along with potassium supplements. Salt-poor albumin will assist with hypoalbuminemia. An esophageal tamponade tube will provide compression of *BLEEDING* on esophageal *VARICES*. Prevent bleeding by soft, nonirritating foods. Let's not give him hot coffee to drink. *LABS* such as liver enzymes will be increased. Hypoalbuminemia, prolonged PT, and altered bilirubin metabolism will be seen in lab reports. Hepatic *ENCEPHALOPATHY* will result if Larry is unable to detoxify ammonia, the end product of protein metabolism. As waste products back up, Larry's *SKIN* will turn jaundiced. Decrease discomfort from pruritus. IS THERE HELP? Avoid cocktails and avoid over-the-counter drugs. Larry's liver is simply unable to detoxify them!

CIRRHOSIS

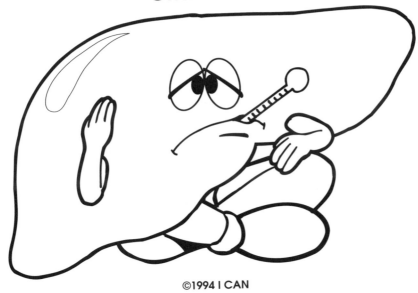

©1994 I CAN

Airway

Swelling

vari**C**es

Inspect lab work

To prevent bleeding

Encephalopathy

Skin

TYLENOL (ACETAMINOPHEN) OVERDOSE

A major undesirable effect of tylenol overdose is hepatic necrosis. It is like we have taken a hammer and beaten "the hell out of the liver." The dose of tylenol should not exceed 4g / day. Other side effects are negligible with recommended dosage. With acute poisoning, the following adverse effects may occur: **anorexia, nausea and vomiting, epigastric or abdominal pain, HEPATOTOXICITY, hypoglycemia, and hepatic coma.**

Tylenol (Acetaminophen) is a very useful drug for pain and fever. (Refer to Poison Control for more specific plans.)

Remember–Do not administer to clients with liver disease.

TYLENOL OVERDOSE

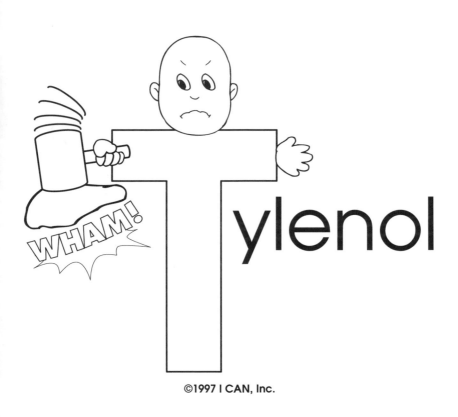

PANCREATITIS

After reviewing the exquisite lips on PAN AM, we feel confident that you will remember the that serum **amylase** and **lipase** are elevated in pancreatitis. **"Pancreas"** will assist you in reviewing the management for these clients.

P *PAIN MANAGEMENT* - Nonnarcotic analgesics (aspirin, ibuprofen, acetaminophen) may be tried. *PANCREATIC ENZYME* repalcement therapy may be indicated.

A *ABDOMINAL PAIN* - Typically, acute pancreatitis produces constant epigastric, periumbilical, or left or right upper abdominal pain radiating to the back, often increased by food and decreased by upright posture. Abdominal tenderness, decreased bowel sounds, distention, and fever may be part of the assessment.

N *NPO* initially - Nasogastric suction for exacerbations, Total Parental Nutrition (TPN) and fluid replacement as necessary. Initiate dietary and insulin therapy for diabetes mellitus secondary to pancreatic insufficiency.

C *CALCIUM* may be low.

R *RISK FACTORS* - Alcoholism, biliary tract disease, a penetrating duodenal ulcer and trauma are also associated with pancreatitis.

E *EVALUATE* glucose, electrolytes, hematocrit, serum amylase and lipase, hypotension, and bowel function.

A *ANALGESICS, ANTICHOLINERGICS, ANTACIDS, H2-receptor ANTAGONISTS, AND ANTIBIOTICS* are utilized.

S *STIMULANTS* such as spices, alcohol, or coffee should be avoided.

PAN AM LIPS

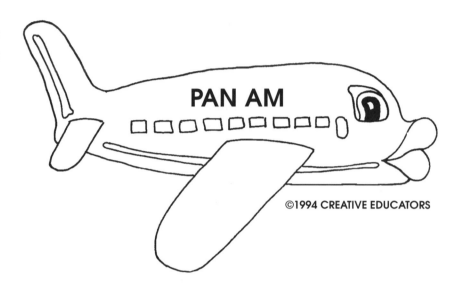

PAN AM

©1994 CREATIVE EDUCATORS

IN PANCREATITIS, AMYLASE AND LIPASE FLY HIGH

MENINGOCELE /
OMPHALOCELE

Both of these disorders have a sac on the outside of the body. The meningocele is a sac-like cyst of meninges filled with spinal fluid that protrudes through a defect in the bony part of the spine. A myelomeningocele is a sac-like cyst containing meninges, spinal fluid and a portion of the spinal cord with its nerves that protrudes through a defect in the vertebral column. The omphalocele is a protrusion of the intestines on the abdomen.

The nursing care is similar to a seal (**CELE**) in the water. We certainly do not want these sacs (**CELES**) to get too dry. Sterile, normal saline soaks may be used to prevent drying.

Correct positioning is also of paramount importance in preventing damage to the sac (**CELE**) as well as providing nursing care after surgery.

**BE KIND TO NATURE AND
KEEP THE SEALS IN THE WATER.**

Meningo<u>CELE</u>/Omphalo<u>CELE</u>

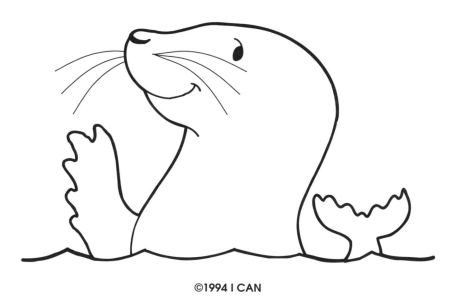

©1994 I CAN

PIES (HYDROCEPHALUS)

Hydrocephalus is caused by an imbalance in the production and absorption of cerebral spinal fluid (CSF) in the ventricles of the brain. This infant will present with an enlarged head. Visualize **PIES** as we refer to the assessments and plans for this condition.

P *PROJECTILE VOMITING* – A symptom of increased intracranial pressure (IICP). Teach parents signs of IICP. Many of these infants are difficult to feed, so small feedings at frequent intervals are recommended.

I *IRRITABILITY* – High pitched cry is characteristic of IICP with an infant. Evaluate the level of consciousness; it is frequently the initial symptom of IICP.

E *ENLARGED HEAD AND FONTANEL* – Normally at birth, the occipital frontal circumference (OFC) is approximately 2–3 cm. larger than the chest circumference. A bulging fontanel is also a sign of IICP.
   EDUCATE family and refer to appropriate community agencies.

S *SEPARATION OF SKULL* – As the CSF increases in the ventricles, there will be a separation of the cranial suture lines. They may have bulging "sunset eyes".
   If infant has a *SHUNT*, observe for infection and IICP.

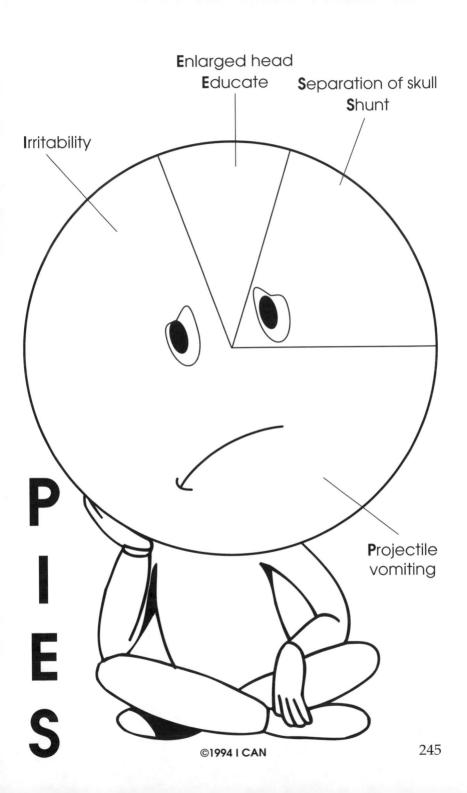

Enlarged head
Educate

Separation of skull
Shunt

Irritability

Projectile
vomiting

P
I
E
S

245

NEUROLOGICAL CHECKS

There has been a lot of mystery around "neuro checks." The bottom line here is that the client remains alert and oriented, the pupils are equal and reactive to light, and all extremities can move on command. Of course, you want to compare with the last time the neuro checks were done. Were the pupils equal and reactive to light? Were all extremities moving spontaneously and to command? PERL MAE is just lying there in her oyster with one side waving her arm and leg while the other side is limp. Observe that one of her pupils is larger than the other.

These assessments are crucial for any neurological client. Observe the subtle differences! For example, is the client more difficult to arouse than earlier? Your response to this change in assessments can mean the difference between a successful or an unsuccessful recovery!

PERL MAE
Pupils Equal Reactive to Light
Moving All Extremities to command

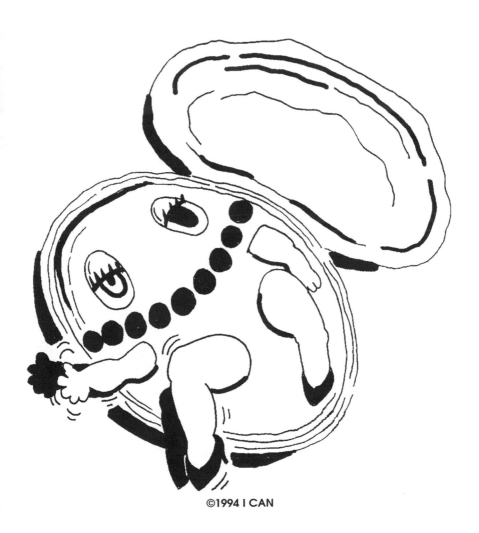

©1994 I CAN

GLASGOW COMA SCALE

GLASGOW COMA SCALE is often found on both nursing exams and physician orders. In the past this scale has been hard to remember, but here's help. Notice that Glasgow is running (a motor runs, indicating MOTOR movements in the client). See Glasgow's EYES are open (the client can open eyes on command). The VERBAL indicator, like the newspaper comics, lets you know that Glasgow is talking (the client has clear verbal ability).

The score for this scale may range from 3–15. The less responsive, the lower the score; the more responsive, the higher the score.

This is a great scale to evaluate the client's level of consciousness! In summary, the Glasgow Coma Scale evaluates motor, eye opening, and verbal ability.

GLASGOW COMA SCALE

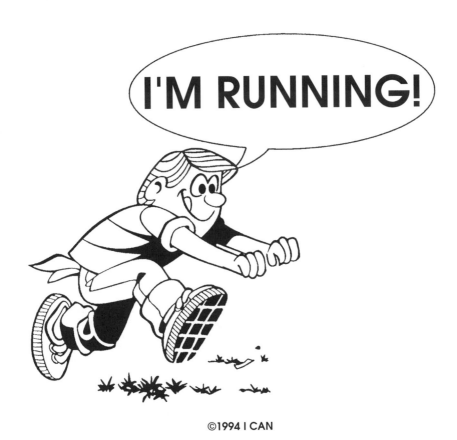

©1994 I CAN

1. MOTOR
2. VERBAL
3. EYES OPEN

VITAL SIGNS FOR SHOCK vs. IICP

Most of us have had the vital signs of shock drilled into our heads. We just have a hard time remembering how those vital signs change with increased intracranial pressure (IICP). Guess what? Vital signs in IICP change exactly opposite to changes in shock. All you have to remember are the vital sign changes in shock and you have the connection to recall the vital sign changes for IICP. Both shock and IICP have one commonality–both cause a loss of consciousness.

VITAL SIGNS FOR SHOCK VS. IICP

Shock	Vs.	IICP
↓	B/P	↑
↑	Pulse	↓
↑	Resp	↓
↓	Temp	↑
↓	Pulse Press	↑
↓	**LOC**	↓

NURSING CARE FOR INCREASED INTRACRANIAL PRESSURE

Nursing care for the clients with increased intracranial pressure is focused on decreasing the pressure and assessing the level of consciousness. For this reason we use the image of a **HEAD** as a memory tool.

H *HOB*–Maintain semi-Fowler's position to promote venous drainage and respiratory function. This would be contraindicated if the client had a spinal cord injury.

E *EVALUATE NEUROLOGICAL CHECKS*–The first sign of a change in the level of intracranial pressure is an alteration in the level of consciousness. Pupils also should react equally to light.

A *AIRWAY*–Evaluate current respiratory pattern. May require intubation and control on a volume ventilator.

D *DRAINAGE*–Drainage from the ears may be cerebral spinal fluid. A CSF leak would test positive for glucose. Apply a sterile dressing over ear and evaluate for signs of meningitis.

S *SAFETY*–Seizure precautions. No sedatives or narcotics. Restrict fluids. Control temperature, and avoid coughing.

NURSING CARE FOR ↑ I C P

HO B—semi-Fowler's

Evaluate ICP

Airway

Drainage

Safety

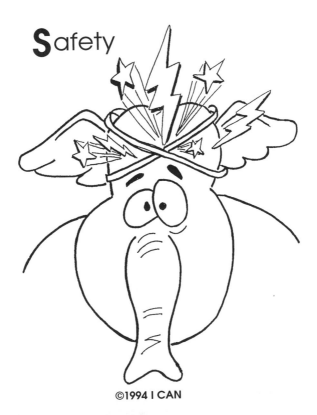

SEIZURES

Caesar is experiencing an interruption of normal brain functioning by uncontrolled paroxysmal discharge of electrical stimuli from the neurons. **"CAESAR"** will outline the general nursing care for clients with seizures.

C *COUNSELING* is important for the family and the client to assist them in maintaining positive coping mechanisms. *CALM* - After a seizure occurs, maintain a calm atmosphere and provide privacy.

A *ANTICONVULSANTS* - Phenobarbital (Sodium luminal), Primidone (Mysoline), Carbamazepine (Tegretol), or Phenytoin (Dilantin) are some examples of anticonvulsants. *APNEA* and / or cyanosis must be monitored. Do not force anything into the client's mouth if the jaws are clenched shut. If the jaws are not clenched, place an airway in the client's mouth after the seizure. Artificial ventilation cannot be performed on a client during a tonic-clonic seizure.

E *EVALUATE* changes in the level of consciousness. After the seizure, evaluate client's orientation, activity, and any level of paralysis or muscle weakness.

S *SAFETY* - Protect the client from injuring himself by falling out of bed or striking himself on bedrails, etc. Loosen any constrictive clothing. Do not restrain client during seizure activity.

A *AVOID ALCOHOL.*
ACTIVITIES - Identify any activities that occurred immediately prior to the seizure. Describe any activity (movement) that occurred and body area affected.

R *REDUCE STIMULI.*
REMAIN with the client who is in seizure activity. Note the time the seizure began and how long it lasted. *REORIENT* client after the seizure.

Remember—SAFETY is the biggest issue.

CAESAR
(SEIZURES)

C
A
E
S
A
R

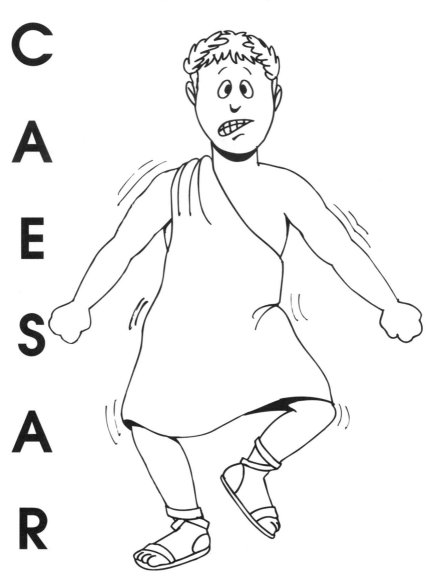

DILANTIN (DIAL AT TEN)

Dilane has a seizure disorder and is taking the drug dilantin. She does not feel well and is calling the nurse at 10:00 a.m. Her therapeutic level for Dilantin should be 10-20 micrograms/ml. (EASY TO REMEMBER. THERE IS A TIN (TEN) IN DILANTIN.) Her adverse reactions from this medication include **gingival hyperplasia,** (see, she's showing you her big gums) **GI disturbances, hepatotoxicity,** (her liver is visible on her abdomen) **ataxia** (her legs are shaking), **hypocalcemia** and a decrease in the absorption of **vitamin D** (the milk on the table and the sunshine coming through the window will help this problem).

If Dilane's level becomes toxic be sure and inform the physician. The medication will likely be decreased.

Remember–Teach good oral hygiene and nutrition.

DILANTIN
(DIAL AT TEN)

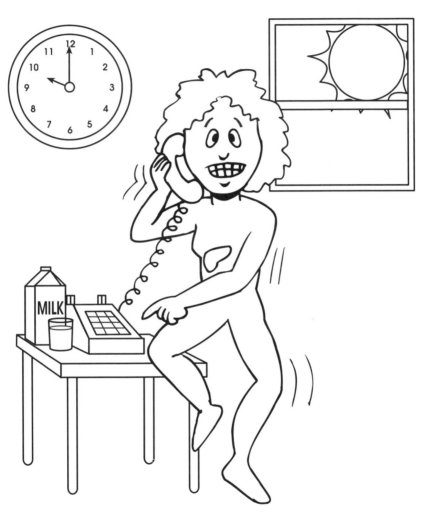

©1997 I CAN, Inc.

PARKINSON'S DISEASE

Meet **PARK DARK**, our little old man with Parkinson's disease. This condition results from a depletion of, or an imbalance in dopamine and increased activity in acetylcholine.

PARK'S fingers want to *"PILL ROLL"* all the time. This tremor is rhythmic and rapid. Worse still, when he gets up out of the chair, his bottom is always trying to catch up with his head and never quite makes it, so he is often *ABOUT TO FALL*. *RIGIDITY* of the muscles results in jerky, uncoordinated "cogwheel" movements. Park is not always the fellow who wants to go to the restaurant for dinner because he *"KAN'T" SWALLOW WELL*, DROOLS his food and might get choked.

Park's last name is **DARK** because this is a dark, depressing disease, and he gets very sad about the whole thing. Medications used to enhance *DOPAMINE* secretion are levodopa (L-DOPA) and SINEMET. *ARTANE* and cogentin are used to decrease effects of acetylcholine. Sometimes *COFFEE RESTRICTION* can reduce the pill rolling. Some ANTIHISTAMINES may be helpful to *KEEP MUSCLE TREMORS DOWN*.

PARK DARK bears watching. He unfortunately falls, spills hot food on himself and can get depressed to the point of harming himself. *He will need your support!*

PARK DARK

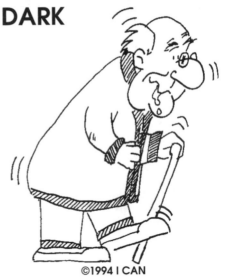

©1994 I CAN

Pill rolling

About to fall

Rigidity

Kan't swallow/speak (drools)

Dopamine/L-Dopa/Sinemet

Artane—improves rigidity

Restrict coffee

Keep tremors down with antihistimine

MYASTHENIA GRAVIS

Why didn't somebody tell us that myasthenia gravis means grave muscle weakness? If they had, we would have asked ourselves where are the muscles? The heart is a muscle. Muscles help move the chest for breathing and the legs for walking, to name just a few. If there is grave muscle weakness, we can see why MYRA DYSTONIA will get into deep trouble fast if she doesn't get her muscle strengthening medication (prostigmin or mestinon) on TIME! As you can see MYRA DYSTONIA has drooping eyelids and may even experience some difficulty moving her face. She will NOT have any sensory deficit, loss of reflexes, or muscle atrophy. This progressive weakness is caused from a failure in transmission of nerve impulses due to acetylcholine release. There are no cures at the present time. **"TIME"** is one of the most important factors.

T *TENSILON* is a drug with a short half life that will strengthen muscle weakness in Myra. This makes it a good drug for DIAGNOSIS and differentiating types of crisis (cholinergic crisis versus myasthenic crisis). It is not routinely given for treatment due to its short term effect.

I *INFECTION* and exercise make MYRA worse.

M *MUST* give medications on time. We sure don't want MYRA to go on that ventilator. We MUST avoid the use of sedatives and tranquilizers which cause respiratory depression. We MUST not give the client anything to eat or drink during a myasthenic crisis due to the risk of aspiration. After the crisis, remember to assess the ability to swallow and give a diet which is soft and easily swallowed.

E *EXACERBATIONS* and remission are part of this experience, but since the weakness is progressive it's likely to get worse with TIME.

MYRA DYSTONIA

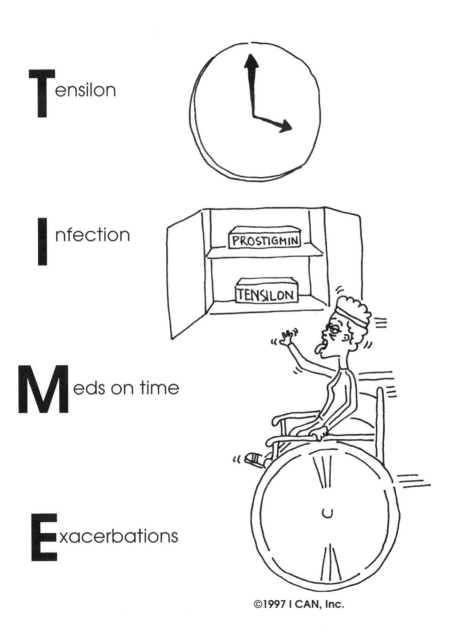

Tensilon

Infection

Meds on time

Exacerbations

BELL'S PALSY

Ring the Bell for the Palsy that affects the seventh cranial nerve, resulting in muscle flaccidity on one side of the face. If the facial appearance is permanent, clients may need counseling assistance with maintaining a *POSITIVE IMAGE*. They may be ringing your call bell because of "**PAINE**" behind the ear, drooping of the mouth and an eyelid that won't close. *ANALGESICS* will be given to decrease the pain behind the ear. Ophthalmic ointment and eye patches may be needed at *NIGHT* to prevent drying of the cornea on the affected side. During the day, *INSTILLING* methylcellulose drops will help keep the eye moist. Due to the discomfort, *EVALUATE* the client's *ABILITY TO EAT*.

Treatment may consist of corticosteroids and vasodilators. An inability to close the eyelid on the affected side, and a sagging mouth is scary; however, proper treatment and good nursing care will usually help clear up the problem with little residual.

BELL'S PALSY

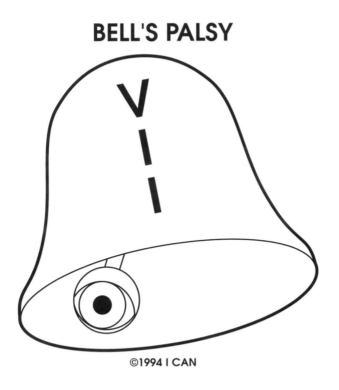

©1994 I CAN

Positive image

Analgesics to decrease pain

Instill methylcellulose drops

Night—opthalmic ointment and eye patches

Evaluate ability to eat

263

TRIGEMINAL NEURALGIA

This is a cranial nerve disorder affecting the sensory branches of the trigeminal nerve (cranial nerve V). Let us introduce you to Luke W. Arm. Luke says, "Hot food is painful!" He has a closed eye from frequent blinking and tearing. Facial twitching and grimacing are characteristic. The pain he experiences is usually brief and ends as abruptly as it begins. The word "**NEURALGIA**" will help you remember the nursing care for Luke W. Arm.

The medical management of pain may be Dilantin or Tegretol. The surgical intervention is a local nerve block or interruption of the nerve impulse transmission.

TRIGEMINAL NEURALGIA

N ature of pain

E ye care

U naffected side—chew on

R oom temperature

A ssess nature of pain

L ukewarm food

hy **G** iene— oral

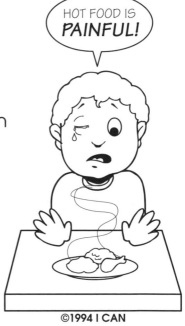

©1994 I CAN

I ncrease protein and calories

A void touching client

ADVERSE EFFECTS OF IMMOBILITY

It is **AWFUL** being immobilized! Have you ever tried it? The nursing goals are to prevent these potential complications from occurring.

A   *ATELECTASIS*–There may be a decrease in client's ability to cough and move those secretions which will result in a decreased oxygen exchange. Infections can lead to this complication. Encourage turning, coughing and deep breathing. Putting the head of the bed up will help with breathing and coughing. Maintain adequate hydration.

W   *WASTING OF THE BONES*–Demineralization of bones leads to muscle weakness and atrophy. Range of motion exercises are mandatory. Maintain appropriate alignment while positioning.

F   *FUNCTION LOSS*–This can result from the above problem. Prevent by active contracting and relaxing large muscles.

U   *URINARY STASIS*–Increase those fluids and decrease the calcium intake. If possible, have client sit to void.

L   *LAST BUT NOT LEAST CONSTIPATION*– Encourage diet with adequate protein, bulk and liquids.

IMMOBILITY

Atelectasis

Wasting of bones

Functional loss of muscle

Urinary stasis

Last but not least, constipation

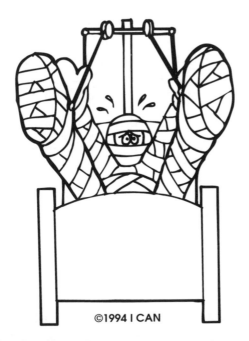

©1994 I CAN

ALLOPURINOL (ZYLOPRIM)

Allopurinol (Zyloprim) the drug of choice to prevent GOUT decreases uric acid synthesis. Uric acid is the end product of purine metabolism. Condition of hyperuricemia may also occur in individuals receiving chemotherapy (secondary gout). Medications for an acute attack may include colchicine, indomethacin (Indocin) or naproxen (Naprosyn).

Gout is generally rapid with swelling and a painful joint. Typically the uric acid crystals are in the large toe, but may also involve ankles and knees. During an acute attack, protect the affected joint by immobilizing the joint. Encourage gradual weight reduction. Instruct the client to avoid salicylates. Encourage **high fluid intake** (>3L / day) to increase excretion of uric acid and to prevent the development of uric acid stones.

Teach clients to avoid foods high in purines such as **organ meats**, shell fish, and preserved fish (anchovies, sardines) and avoid **alcohol**. We would like to see the urine **output increased** to 2 liters per day to help decrease the risk of stones. Clients at risk for stones may be given trisodium citrate for urine alkalinization.

Remember–Clients with renal insufficiency should receive a reduced dose of Allopurinol.

ALLOPURINOL (GOUT)

Gulp 3 liters fluid per day

Ø organ meats or wines

Urine output increased to 2 liters per day

Teach

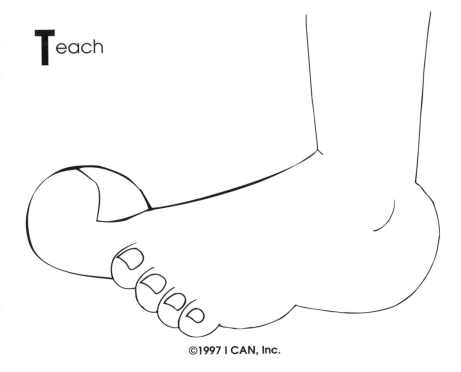

©1997 I CAN, Inc.

OSTEOPOROSIS

JOSEPHINE BONE-A-PART is working to prevent immobility in her "mature years". She is on a treadmill because weight-bearing exercise increases bone strength. She is taking her Fosomax, Calcium, and Estrogen to decrease her risk of developing osteoporosis. She knows that her drinking and smoking have got to stop if she doesn't want to be laid up with broken **BONES**.

B   *BONE* density studies are the noninvasive x-ray diagnostic tests that are commonly used. There is no prep, no pain and not much time involved in this x-ray. Just lie down and they'll shoot it.

O   *OUT* of calcium is an issue. Inadequate calcium intake early in life may have predisposed Josephine Bone-A-Part to the development of osteoporosis. Calcium supplemental therapy (about 1500mg per day) is usually recommended for post-menopausal women. Young women should be advised to have a daily dietary intake of at least 1000 to 1500 mg of calcium per day. Magnesium and Vitamin D may also need to be supplemented.

N   *NEED FOSOMAX* **AFTER** osteoporosis has developed. This drug aides the BONES to become more calcified, stronger and denser. To keep down the GI side effects of this medication, drink with 8 ounces of water first thing in the morning. Stay sitting up and NPO for at least half an hour before eating or taking other drugs. Yep, it's a pain!

E   *ESTROGEN* given orally has demonstrated its ability to decrease the incidence of osteoporosis. In addition, estrogen improves the client's lipid profile (HDL cholesterol rises, LDL cholesterol falls) and overall cardiovascular risk declines. Weight bearing EXERCISE, such as walking, helps the BONES. EDUCATION early in life will assist in preventing complications from osteoporosis.

S   *STRESS* fractures especially of the hip, waist or vertebra are common. Education and prevention of falls are important in minimizng fractures and maintaining independence for post-menopausal women.

Remember—Prevention is the BEST action!

JOSEPHINE BONE-A-PART

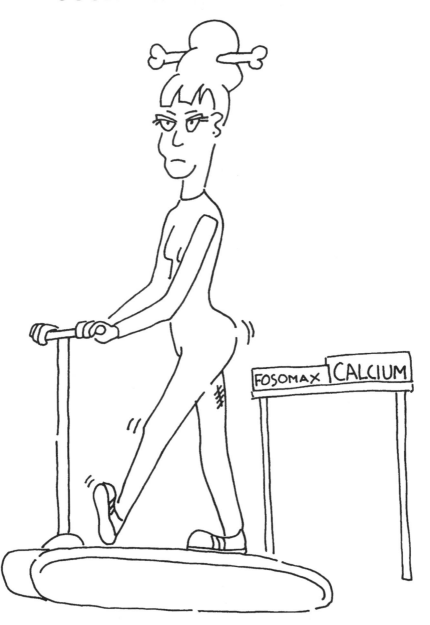

ARTHRITIS

Arthur has osteoarthritis. He wakes up in the morning stiff and achy and finds it hard to reach his walking cane. His fingers are all swollen at the joints (Herberden's nodules) and other joints are affected. He may feel better after his shower as the hot water warms up those joints. Arthur has on his swim trunks because he is going to water therapy at the local spa. Water therapy is probably the best exercise since it better protects his weight bearing joints. He will definitely need to rest after his swim.

Tylenol may be the medication of choice and Arthur will have to be reminded to keep his dosage at or below 4 gms/24 hours to prevent an overdose. (See TYLENOL OVERDOSE)

Remember–Arthur may not want to move because of his pain, but physical activity is imperative for him to retain his independence.

ARTHUR ITIS

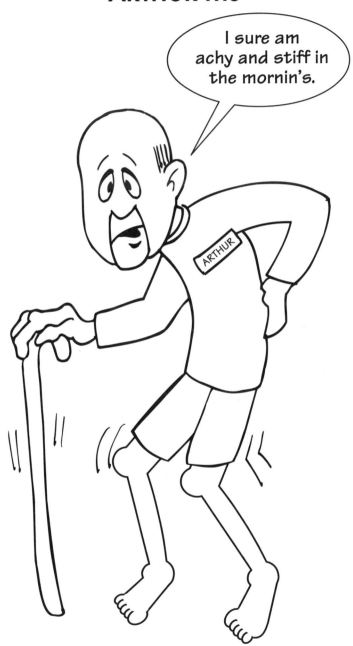

NONSTEROIDAL ANTI-INFLAMMATORY DRUGS (NSAIDs)

NSAIDs are a group of medications that prevent prostaglandin synthesis. What does that mean? Prostaglandins contribute to the following: inflammation, body temperature, pain transmission, platelett aggregation, and other actions. These prostaglandins are not stored, but are released on demand.

What type of physical problems may benefit from NSAIDs? Fever and inflammation (ie. arthritis) can be reduced by these medications.

Are there any undesirable effects from NSAIDs? There are several undesirable effects that the nurse must assess and educate clients to report. These include GI upset or bleeding, **ototoxicity** (ringing in the ears), **hepatic necrosis**, or **nephritis**.

As a nurse, what should be included in the plan of care?

1. Administer medications with **food to decrease GI irritation.**

2. Teach clients about actions and side effects and report any dark, tarry stools, "coffee ground or bloody emesis", other **GI distress** or **ringing in the ears.**

3. Instruct client to inform health care providers about these medications prior to any dental or other type of surgery. NSAIDs should be discontinued approximately 7 days before the procedure to prevent any complications with bleeding.

4. NSAIDs are not the drugs of choice if the client has any compromise in either the renal system or the liver.

5. Evaluate the effectiveness of the NSAIDs.

NSAIDs

N aprosyn

S ulindac (Clinoril)

A leve
naprox

I buprofen
ndocin

D o take with food
olobid

S alicylates

CARE OF CLIENT IN TRACTION

Ellie Elephant gets in more trouble. She has fallen, **FRAC-TURED** her trunk, and is in traction. We will need a *FIRM MATTRESS*, and will probably need help putting her through *RANGE OF MOTION* exercises. Pay attention to those feet; we don't want a problem with *FOOT DROP*. Without good body *ALIGNMENT*, Ellie may get contractures and decubiti. *ALIGNMENT* will also help keep the traction pulling from both ends which is the reason for traction anyway. Let's get Ellie a *TRAPEZE*, so that she can help us turn her to keep the pneumonia away. Ellie needs to cough and deep breathe on regular intervals to prevent *RESPIRATORY COMPLICA-TIONS*. One *COMPLICATION* of a fracture of long bones is a fat embolism. It can be transported to the lungs producing symptoms of acute *RESPIRATORY* distress. Now what will we do about her *URINARY RETENTION*? Increase fluid intake. Ellie may need help with the bedpan. Be sure and *EVALUATE FOR CIRCULATORY IMPAIRMENTS*. The 5 P's will help. They are pain, pallor of skin, pulses (especially distal to the injury), paresthesia, and paralysis. Compartmental syndrome can be a major problem.

Good Luck! Elephants and people in traction can be a major challenge!

CARE OF CLIENT IN TRACTION

F irm mattress
F oot drop

R OM—for unaffected
    extremities

A lignment

C omplications

T rapeze

U rinary retention

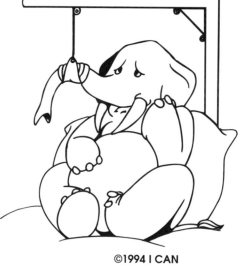

©1994 I CAN

R espiratory complications

E valuate circulatory
    impairments
        (5 P's)

CARE OF THE SPINAL CORD CLIENT

"**CRUTCHES** THE COLLIE" dog has been out partying with the neighborhood dogs and has been in an automobile accident. He broke his neck and is unfortunately paralyzed from the neck down. The paramedic dog who came to the scene had to access his airway by a "jaw thrust" and log roll him to stabilize his neck. This will minimize further *CORD DAMAGE*. Assess Collie's breath sounds and signs of hypoxia. Incentive spirometry and chest physiotherapy will assist in optimizing *RESPIRATORY FUNCTION*. Due to his loss of bladder function, *URINARY* retention is a problem. He will either have an indwelling catheter or require intermittent catheterization. Prevent urinary tract infections! Because Collie is immobile watch for blood clots (*THROMBUS*). Compression stockings may help venous return. *CARDIOVASCULAR STABILITY* can be a problem due to *SHOCK* or autonomic dysreflexia. (Refer to **Autonomic Dysreflexia**.)

Collie needs a *NEURO ASSESSMENT* for IICP (Refer to IICP visual). *FLUIDS AND ROUGHAGE* are necessary to keep bladder and bowels working. Calories and protein need to be increased. Watch for *SKIN BREAKDOWN*. An ounce of prevention is worth a pound of cure. Collie is going to have a major life change. He will need *SUPPORT* in ventilating his feelings and establishing realistic short-term goals.

CARE OF SPINAL CORD CLIENT

Cord damage

Respiratory function

Urinary and bowel function

Thrombus

Cardiovascular stability

Help maintain ongoing
    neurological assessment

Encourage adequate
    fluid and nutrition

kin breakdown
Shock
upport

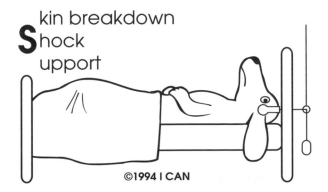

©1994 I CAN

ANTICOAGULANTS

Coumadin and Heparin are used to inhibit thrombus and clot formation. They chip away at the clot to make it smaller. Clotting times will be prolonged which will assist in maintaining the flow or "stream of blood."

The key to successfully remembering the lab reports and antidotes for the appropriate anticoagulants are to think of (H) looking like 2 tt's in Heparin. The lab report necessary to evaluate while clients are on heparin is Ptt. The antidote also has 2 t's in it (protamine sulfate).

Coumadin's antidote is vitamin K. **C** and **K** sound alike which will help with association. The lab report which needs to be monitored is Pt.

Labs now report INR (international normalized ratio) values. The range for most clients on anticoagulants is 2–3. The exceptions are mechanical heart valves and recurrent thromboembolism clients who should be anticoagulated to an INR of 3–4.5.

ANTICOAGULANTS

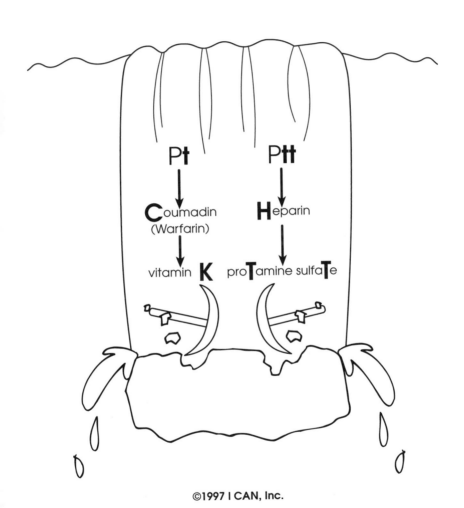

AUTONOMIC DYSREFLEXIA

This condition may occur in clients with a spinal cord injury at T-6 or higher. The stimuli below the level of injury triggers the sympathetic nervous system to dump catecholamines resulting in hypertension. Spinal injury blocks the normal transmission of sensory impulses. There is an exaggerated response to the sensory stimuli.

The most common causes are the **3 F's**: *FULL BLADDER, FECAL IMPACTION*, and a *FUNNY FEELING WITH THE SKIN*.

The assessments that occur as a result of these causes are: FLUSHING, and DIAPHORESIS, HEADACHE, HYPERTEN-SION, and BRADYCARDIA. The priority treatment is to identify and REMOVE the CAUSE. Frequently the dysreflexia will subside. If possible, the head of the bed can be elevated. Watch the hypertension, so that it doesn't get out of hand.

These folks feel real bad and usually cannot tell you their problem. Once their bladder or bowel is emptied the sweating and bad feelings go away.

AUTONOMIC DYSREFLEXIA
(Injuries at T_6 or higher)

Causes

1. **F**ull bladder
2. **F**ecal impaction
3. **F**unny feeling with the skin

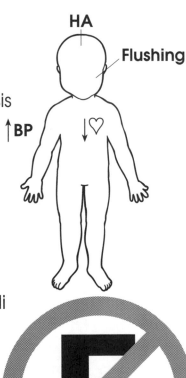

Assessments

1. Flushing & Diaphoresis
2. Headache
3. Hypertension
4. Bradycardia

Plan

Remove noxious stimuli

MAGIC 2s

The magician is pulling the prescription drugs out of his magic hat and reminding you that you can use the"MAGIC 2s"as a way to remember the toxicity level. These are the medications most commonly monitored for therapeutic dosage.

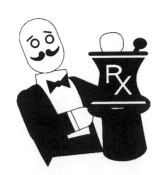

Monitoring Drugs
By The Magic 2s

Drug	Range	Toxicity
Digitalis	.5-1.5	**2**
Lithium	.6-1.2	**2**
Aminophylline (Theophylline)	10-20	**20**
Dilantin	10-20	**20**
Acetaminophen	1-30	**200**

ELECTROLYTE MAGIC

Sometimes it's hard to remember those electrolyte extracellular levels; however, we MUST because they affect the heart as recorded by the EKG. The digit 4 can be magic in helping to remember. Even though not electrolytes, the hemoglobin and hematocrit can also be remembered using a 4. For example if the hemoglobin is 14 the hematocrit will be 42.

Electrolyte Magic
Remember the 4s

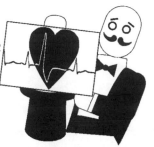

Electrolyte	Range	Magic 4
K	3.5-5.5	4
CO_2	23-30	24
Cl	98-106	104
Na	135-145	140

A good way to remember the Hct is: 3 x Hb (10-14)

COST RANGE OF MEDICATIONS

This cost range list is inconclusive and includes only those medications reviewed throughout this book. This list serves as a reference for the ranges of price per dose.

$	generally under $.25 per dose
$$	range from $.26-$1.00 per dose
$$$	range from $1.01-$2.00 per dose
$$$$	range from $2.01-$3.00 per dose
$$$$$	range from $3.01-$10.00 per dose
$	megabucks! over $100.00 per dose

ANALGESICS

Acetaminophen	$
Aleve	$
Anaprox	$$$
Aspirin	$
Ibuprofen	$
Indocin	$
Naprosyn	$$
Sulindac	$$

ANTACIDS

Amphogel	$$
Maalox	$
Mylanta	$
Riopan	$
Rolaids	$
Titralac	$

ANTIBIOTICS

Gentamycin	$$
Neomycin	$$
Streptomycin	$$
Tetracycline	$

ANTICHOLINERGICS

Atropine .... $$
Banthine .... $$
Bentyl .... $$
Pro-Banthine .... $$

ANTICOAGULANTS

Coumadin .... $$
Heparin .... $$

ANTICONVULSANTS

Dilantin... $
Phenobarbital .... $
Tegretol .... $

ANTIDEPRESSANTS

(Tricyclics)
　　Aventyl .... $$
　　Elavil .... $
　　Norpramin .... $$
　　Sinequan.. $
　　Tofranil .... $
　　Vivactil... $$

(Monoamine Oxide Inhibitors)
　　Marplan... $$
　　Nardil .... $$
　　Parnate .... $$

ANTIFUNGAL

Amphotericin .... *$*

ANTIHYPERTENSIVES

(Ace Inhibitors)
　　Altace... $$
　　Capoten .... $

Monopril .... $$
Vasotec .... $$

(Beta Blockers)
Corgard .... $$
Inderal .... $
Lopressor .... $$
Tenormin .... $
Visken .... $$

(Calcium Channel Blockers)
Cardene .... $$
Cardizem .... $$$
Plendil .... $$
Procardia .... $$$
Isoptin .... $$

(Adrenergic Blocking Agents)
Aldomet .... $
Catapres .... $$

ANTIMANIC
Lithium .... $

ANTIPARKINSONIAN
Artane .... $
Cogentin .... $
Eldepryl .... $$$$
Parlodel .... $$$
Permax .... $$
Symmetrel .... $$

ANTITUBERCULIN AGENTS
Ethambutol .... $
Isoniazid .... $
Rifampin .... $

Streptomycin ....$

ANXIOLYTIC AGENTS

Atarax ....$
Equanil ....$
Librium ....$
Serax...$
Valium ....$

BRONCHODILATORS

Adrenalin ....$$$$$
Proventil ....$$
Theo-Dur ....$$
Ventolin ....$$

CORTICOSTEROIDS

Aerobid...$$
Azmacort..$$
Decadron ....$$

DIURETICS

Aldactone ....$$
Edecrin...$$
Hydrodiuril...$
Lasix ....$

EXPECTORANTS

Robitussin ....$

GOUT

Allopurinol ....$

HISTAMINE H2-BLOCKERS

Axid .... $$$
Pepcid ....$$
Tagament ....$$$

Zantac .... $$

INSULIN
Humalog .... $$
Lente .... $
NPH .... $
Regular .... $
Semilente .... $
Ultralente .... $

NSAIDs
(Refer to Analgesics)

OPHTHALAMIC AGENTS
Atropine .... $
Carbachol .... $
Carpine .... $
Cyclogyl .... $
Epinephrine .... $
Mydriacyl .... $
Pilocarpine .... $

OSTEOPOROSIS
Calcium Supplements .... $
Fosomax .... $$$

THYROID REPLACEMENT
Synthroid... $

Notes for Bright Ideas

"It's all right to have butterflies in your stomach. Just get them to fly in formation."
Dr. Rob Gilbert

Notes for Bright Ideas

"If you believe you can or you can't,
you're right."

Marge Cooper

Notes for Bright Ideas

"Surround yourself with people who respect and treat you well."

Claudia Black

INDEX

Note: Page numbers in italics refer to images.

—A—

People learn in many different ways. We want to tell you about our stuff because our business is to help you PASS.

NURSING MADE INSANELY EASY, 2nd Ed. is a pocket-sized book, chock full of drawings and information streamlining nursing and allied health education with an EASY totally different bottom line approach to concepts.

- E   essential concepts assist learners to prepare for exams and NCLEX.
- A   assist nursing graduates to remember health and disease concepts.
- S   special images per page with essential concepts on the opposite page.
- Y   your learning is memorable and fun.

For example, one look at "Go Getter Gertrude" and you will remember the most important facts about the concept of hyperthyroidism and Graves' Disease _forever._

NCLEX-RN™: 101 HOW TO PASS 2nd Ed.
Helps you **FOCUS** on your success!

- F   feel more confident
- O   omit surprises on NCLEX-RN™
- C   cut through piles of notes
- U   use to pinpoint your study needs
- S   see yourself improve

The book has over 800 critical thinking questions based on nursing behaviors that are the backbone of the NCLEX-RN™ exam. It comes with a pharmacology disk of 60 items so that you can practice on the computer before "test day".

NCLEX-RN™ REVIEW audio tapes. Pass your NCLEX with confidence after these fun and easy listening audio tapes. These tapes are of an actual live review course that includes the concepts listed in the NCLEX-RN™ test plan. The NURSING MADE INSANELY EASY book comes with this set of 7 tapes. We CAN help you prepare for the NCLEX and you can listen at your convenience!

NCLEX-RN™ non-traditional live review, brought to your site for 50 participants or more or call our office 1-800-234-0575 for information and dates on our sites in more than 15 states. The NCLEX exam did not get harder just different. This course provides the SECRETS to NCLEX success in a fun and easy 4 day format. The book NURSING MADE INSANELY EASY, 2nd ed. and the book NCLEX-RN ™ 101: HOW TO PASS, 2nd ed. with pharmacology disk are included in the cost of this review course.

Order now!

To order call 1-800-234-0575 or mail to ICAN Publishing, Inc. P.O. 1135, Shreveport. LA 71163 or Fax your order to 1-318-686-5094. We accept Mastercard, Visa , Discover cards , money orders or personal checks. Please do not send cash in the mail.

✂ — — — — — — — — — — — — — — — — — — —

Yes, I wish to order:

❏ **NCLEX RN™ 101: HOW TO PASS, 2nd edition** by Rayfield & Manning with pharmacology disk • **$24.95 plus $4.00 shipping and handling**

❏ **NURSING MADE INSANELY EASY, 2nd edition** by Rayfield & Manning • **$24.95 plus $4.00 shipping and handling**

❏ **NCLEX-RN™ Review Cassette Tapes** by Sylvia Rayfield & Associates, Inc. (Includes NURSING MADE INSANELY EASY) • **$124.95 plus $4.00 shipping and handling.**

❏ **Register me for a Sylvia Rayfield & Associates Review Course** • **$230** (Includes NURSING MADE INSANELY EASY, 2nd ed. and NCLEX-RN™ 101: HOW TO PASS, 2nd ed. with pharmacology disk).

Be sure and call to tell us where you want to take the review course. Discounts are given to groups of more than 50 participants!

"The NCLEX-RN™ exam did NOT get harder, just different."

We know if you believe you can pass, you will. We developed these tools to help!